Calorie Counter Journal

FOR

DUMMIES®

by Rosanne Rust, MS, RD, LDN
Meri Raffetto, RD

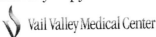
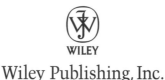

WILEY

Wiley Publishing, Inc.

Calorie Counter Journal For Dummies®

Published by
Wiley Publishing, Inc.
111 River St.
Hoboken, NJ 07030-5774
www.wiley.com

WILEY

Table of Contents

Introduction

*L*osing weight takes time, focus, and effort, and not every-one is genetically predisposed to a flat belly. The magazine ads and Web sites promising to speed up your weight loss are just trying to fool you. Quick fixes don't exist for weight loss, but there is one important tool that can make the process easier — and ultimately make you more successful as you go about it. That tool is a food and exercise journal.

Studies have shown that keeping a food and exercise journal helps individuals achieve successful weight loss. In fact, in one study, participants who kept a food journal four to seven days a week lost an average of 18 pounds compared with an average of 9 pounds lost by the non-journal-keepers. These results suggest that by simply keeping a food journal, you may lose twice the weight than if you don't keep a journal.

Why do food and exercise journals work? Important components of weight-loss intervention include providing account-ability and implementing behavior strategies that modify eating and exercise habits. Keeping a journal helps you pin-point problem areas, make positive changes, and then moni-tor and regulate your habits — all of which helps you stay accountable to yourself (or even your doctor or dietitian). It also helps you target barriers to weight loss. Being aware of problem behaviors and managing them is key to successful weight management over a lifetime.

Journaling can also help you stick with your goals for a longer period of time. Setting short-term goals and using a journal to track your progress toward those goals helps prevent dis-couragement, thereby leading to long-term success.

People have different reasons for wanting to shed pounds. Some are fixated on bathing suit season, whereas others just want to buy smaller pants. Some simply want to look better in their clothes; others feel they need to take control of their health. In the long run, your health is the real reason to be concerned about being overweight. This little book makes it easy to keep track of your eating and exercise. In just minutes a day, it can help you stay motivated and on track with your goals, proving that your good health is worth your time.

About This Book

Calorie Counter Journal For Dummies is a handy record-keeping guide that's chock-full of helpful information such as a quick overview of good nutrition (including sports nutrition) and the steps you need to take to change problem behaviors. We help you set detailed goals that are specific to you and show you how to change up your routine for a healthier one that balances calorie intake with physical activity.

Then of course there's the meat of the book: the food and exercise journal, complete with instructions for how to keep such a journal. Each journal page includes room to record your food and beverage intake, mood, energy level, and exercise details. It also provides space to log your goals and track your weight changes. There are even weekly assessment pages designed to help you take a look at the bigger picture so you can better see positive trends in your behaviors and overall health. What can we say? We want you to get your money's worth and get on the road to good health at the same time.

Conventions Used in This Book

We use the following conventions in this book:

- ✓ **Boldface** helps the key words and phrases in bulleted lists stand out.

- ✓ *Italics* indicate terminology we're defining for you, as well as words we want to emphasize.

- ✓ Monofont lets you know you're looking at a Web site address.

Foolish Assumptions

Calorie Counter Journal For Dummies is for anyone who's interested in improving his or her diet and exercise habits but hasn't been able to figure out where to start. If any of these statements ring true to you, then you've picked up the right book:

✔ You have difficulty losing weight and pinpointing barriers to weight loss.

✔ You've tried to diet, but you can't seem to figure out why you aren't losing weight.

✔ You face challenges with emotional eating (meaning you eat when you aren't hungry simply because you're feeling sad, stressed, or bored).

✔ You have a history of being overweight or obese.

✔ You've hit a plateau in your weight loss (meaning you just can't lose additional weight no matter how hard you try).

✔ You're having trouble maintaining weight loss.

✔ Your doctor or dietitian has instructed you to keep a food and exercise journal.

✔ You're concerned about eating well in order to improve your overall health, control high blood pressure, lower your cholesterol, manage diabetes, or improve your athletic performance.

How This Book Is Organized

Calorie Counter Journal For Dummies is divided into three parts designed to help you set and meet your goals.

Part 1: Setting Goals and Tracking Calories

First off in this part, we give you a nutrition primer to help you make healthy choices; we also show you how to read a food label and determine proper serving sizes. Next, we fill you in on everything you need to know to set achievable goals and get your brain thinking past the almighty scale. (After all, losing weight has repercussions beyond just fitting into smaller jeans.) Finally, we walk you through the process of monitoring and measuring your goals and reveal just how many calories you burn doing different activities.

Part II: How to Use a Food and Exercise Journal

This part helps you begin a food and exercise journal, providing you with samples as well as tips for balancing healthy eating with exercise. If you're an athlete, pay close attention to this part to discover how keeping a journal can help with improving your athletic performance (or with dropping those pounds that keep slowing you down).

Part III: Journal

Part III is where you'll spend much of your time. It's home to the actual journal pages, each of which allows you to customize what you want to record so that your food and exercise journal suits your personal goals.

Icons Used in This Book

Although we consider all the information in this book important to you in your quest to lose weight and live a healthier lifestyle, some of the information is more important than the rest. These paragraphs are marked with one of the following icons.

If you remember nothing else from these pages, you should walk away from this book with a running list of information marked by this icon.

Maintaining a healthy lifestyle is a little easier when you know the information spotlighted by this bull's-eye.

Where to Go from Here

If you need to brush up on nutrition basics or you want to unravel the mystery of portion control, head to Part I. If you want to dive in and write down your first journal entry, go straight to Part III. However, we do suggest you read through Part II before you begin journaling so you can get the most out of your journal. With that said, best of luck on your new road to self-awareness and health!

Part I
Setting Goals and Tracking Calories

The 5th Wave   By Rich Tennant

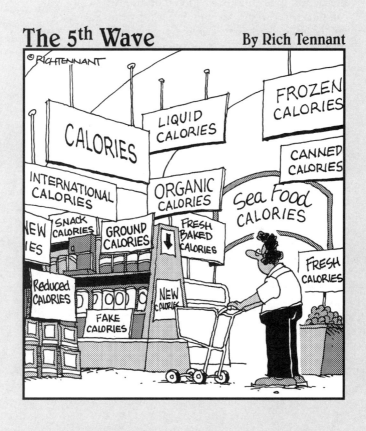

In this part . . .

The whole purpose of keeping a food and exercise journal is to a) help you find a way to meet your diet and health goals and b) keep you on the right track after you find what works for you. Whether you want to lose weight, manage diabetes, lower your blood pressure or cholesterol, or improve your overall health, this part helps you assess your current health and fitness status, determine how many calories you need based on your activity level and whether you're trying to lose or maintain weight, and refresh your memory of nutrition basics.

Part I also helps you figure out where to begin when it comes to changing your lifestyle. You discover how to set detailed goals, monitor your progress toward those goals, and establish a routine. If you're working on weight loss, you'll find loads of tips in this part to help you stay on track. To help you achieve your goals, we give you healthy eating tips, insight into how many calories you burn during various activities, and some ideas for starting an exercise program. Well, what are you waiting for? We think the scale is about to tilt in your favor.

Chapter 1

Getting Started

· ·

In This Chapter

▶ Gauging how healthy you truly are

▶ Calculating how many calories your body requires

▶ Surveying the five food groups

▶ Determining proper serving sizes

· ·

*F*iguring out your body mass index, calorie needs, and general fitness level helps you set the tone for what goals you want to achieve, and improving both your eating habits and your fitness can provide you with the encouragement you need to continue making strides toward better health. That's why this chapter helps you obtain some baseline measurements, sort through the food groups, and understand portion control. With this information, you'll have a solid foundation for getting started on your health and fitness goals.

Assessing Your Current Health Status

Understanding your health status is an important step toward improving your health. The best way to obtain an overview of your health is to have your doctor conduct an annual physical exam.

At a typical physical exam, you can expect to be weighed; have your blood pressure, heart, lungs, and abdominal area checked; be screened for various health risks; and have a chance to chat about any problems you're experiencing. Depending on your medical and family history, your doctor may also draw blood in order to screen it for high cholesterol, diabetes, or other conditions. The information you receive from this visit not only helps you determine your health status but also what you may need to work on (like exercising more, eating fewer high-sodium foods, losing weight, and so on).

Of course, there are other ways of determining your current health status besides paying a visit to your doctor. You can also evaluate your body mass index (BMI), your health risk factors (both controllable and uncontrollable), and your current fitness level. We explain how in the following sections.

Calculating your BMI

One fairly reliable way to assess your health is to take a look at your BMI. *BMI* is an indicator of body fatness; it's calculated from a person's weight and height. Where your number falls on the BMI scale helps you see whether you're underweight, normal weight, overweight, or obese.

- ✔ A normal adult BMI ranges from 18.5 to 24.9.
- ✔ An overweight adult BMI goes from 25 to 29.9.
- ✔ An obese adult BMI is 30 or higher.

Use Table 1-1 to figure out where your BMI falls.

Don't see your numbers in Table 1-1? Access an easy-to-use BMI calculator online at www.reallivingnutrition.com.

The higher your BMI climbs, the greater your risk of developing health problems. If your BMI is 25 or higher, your best bet is to develop a plan to lose weight and then manage your weight loss. A food and exercise journal is an excellent tool to include in your program. Good thing you already picked up this book, huh?

Knowing your risk factors

Several factors affect the state of your current and future health. Some of these factors are controllable, and some aren't. For instance, you don't have control over your genetic makeup (specifically your family history of disease and your race), your gender, or your age, but you do have control over your body weight, whether or not you smoke, your diet, and the amount of exercise you get.

Taking control of the factors that are within your power can lead to improved health and a reduced risk for disease.

Figuring out just how physically fit you are

Assessing your fitness level before you start keeping a food and exercise journal can give you a better understanding of where your physical fitness is at currently and where you want it to go so you can set goals and monitor your progress toward them. Here are some simple ways to assess your fitness level:

✔ **Test your aerobic fitness.** Take a brisk 1-mile walk on a treadmill and check your pulse before and after. Record both pulses and the time in minutes that it took you to walk a mile. A healthy 30- to 60-year-old adult can walk a mile in 13 to 16 minutes with a steady pulse (around 110 to 170 beats per minute).

✔ **See how many push-ups you can do.** Your average healthy guy or gal can do at least five push-ups.

✔ **Test your flexibility.** Sit on the floor with your legs straight in front of you and place a yardstick or measuring tape on the floor between your legs. (The 9-inch mark should be even with the soles of your feet, with the 0 closer to your knees.) Stretch toward your toes and record how far you reached. Do this two more times and note the average distance. A typical male can stretch up to 2 inches on average, and a typical female can stretch anywhere from 0.5 to 4 inches on average. Anything beyond that is considered good to excellent.

✔ **Estimate your body composition.** Calculate your BMI and, using a tape measure, measure your waist circumference at its smallest point. (Keep in mind that today's pant styles are way below a person's actual waist.) A healthy waist measurement for men is less than 40 inches; for women, it's less than 35 inches. To find out what constitutes a good BMI, see the earlier "Calculating your BMI" section.

Based on the results of these fitness tests, you can set goals to improve the fitness area(s) in which you're lacking. (We help you set realistic, achievable goals in Chapter 2.) You can also repeat these tests periodically, such as once a month for four months, in order to monitor how your fitness level has improved since you started keeping your food and exercise journal.

Table 1-1

Body Mass Index

Height	19	20	21	22	23	24	25	26	27	28	29	30	31	32	33	34	35
							Body Weight (Pounds)										
58"	91	96	100	105	110	115	119	124	129	134	138	143	148	153	158	162	167
59"	94	99	104	109	114	119	124	128	133	138	143	148	153	158	163	168	173
60"	97	102	107	112	118	123	128	133	138	143	148	153	158	163	168	174	179
61"	100	106	111	116	122	127	132	137	143	148	153	158	164	169	175	180	185
62"	104	109	115	120	126	131	136	142	147	153	158	164	169	175	180	186	191
63"	107	113	118	124	130	135	141	146	152	158	163	169	175	180	186	191	197
64"	110	116	122	128	134	140	145	151	157	163	169	174	180	186	192	197	204
65"	114	120	126	132	138	144	150	156	162	168	174	180	186	192	198	204	210
66"	118	124	130	136	142	148	155	161	167	173	179	185	192	198	204	210	216
67"	121	127	134	140	146	153	159	166	172	178	185	191	198	204	211	217	223
68"	125	131	138	144	151	158	164	171	177	184	190	197	203	210	216	223	230

69"	128	135	142	149	155	162	169	176	182	189	196	203	209	216	223	230	236
70"	132	139	146	153	160	167	174	181	188	195	202	209	216	222	229	236	243
71"	136	143	150	157	165	172	179	186	193	200	208	215	222	229	236	243	250
72"	140	147	154	162	169	177	184	191	199	206	213	221	228	235	242	250	258
73"	144	151	159	166	174	182	189	197	204	212	219	227	235	242	250	257	265
74"	148	155	163	171	179	186	194	202	210	218	225	233	241	249	256	264	272
75"	152	160	168	176	184	192	200	208	216	224	232	240	248	256	264	272	279
76"	156	164	172	180	189	197	205	213	221	230	238	246	254	263	271	279	287

Source: The National Heart, Lung, and Blood Institute

Determining Your Calorie Needs

A *calorie* is a unit of measurement used to describe how much energy is provided from foods and beverages. To maintain a healthy weight throughout your life, you need to know how many calories you're using and consuming. When you consume more calories than you use, you gain weight. When you consume fewer calories than you use, you lose weight. It's as simple as that. The next sections walk you through what affects your calorie needs and how to calculate your magic number.

The influences

You require different amounts of calories at different stages of your life. Children, teenagers, and pregnant women require greater numbers of calories to support growth, whereas adult men and women have lower calorie needs. Making matters even harder, a person's calorie needs continue to decline with age.

Your individual calorie needs also vary depending on your age, gender, physical activity level, and body composition. As a person ages, his percentage of body fat increases, which results in a lower *basal metabolic rate,* or BMR (which is the amount of calories your body burns at rest for basic functioning). Severely cutting down on your calorie intake also reduces your BMR, but having more lean mass (muscle) than fat helps boost it. Consequently, the best plan is to make smaller decreases in calorie intake while increasing your daily physical activity.

The math

To determine your individual energy needs, we recommend using the *Harris-Benedict Equation.* It's one of the most commonly used equations for calculating *basal energy expenditure,* or BEE (which is interchangeable with BMR). The equation takes into consideration your age, gender, height, and weight. Here are the formulas:

For men:

BEE = 66 + (6.23 × Weight in pounds) + (12.7 × Height in inches) – (6.8 × Age in years)

For women:

BEE = 655 + (4.35 × Weight in pounds) + (4.7 × Height in inches) – (4.7 × Age in years)

Your total calorie requirements equal your BEE multiplied by estimated activity factors of 1.2 (inactive) to 1.9 (very active), depending on your activity level. For example, if your BEE is 1,300 and you exercise 3 to 5 days per week, you'd multiply 1,300 by 1.5 to find that you really need 1,950 calories to maintain your current weight. Table 1-2 helps you figure out which estimated activity factor to multiply your BEE by based on your activity level. (Note that most adult women require about 1,500 to 2,200 calories a day, whereas most adult men require 2,200 to 2,800 calories a day.)

Table 1-2 Activity Factors by Activity Level

Activity Level	Estimated Activity Factor
Sedentary	1.2
Light housework or yardwork, walking around town	1.3
Heavy housework or yardwork	1.4
Regular house chores plus moderate exercise 2 to 3 days per week	1.5
Regular house chores plus moderate exercise 3 to 4 days per week	1.6
Regular house chores plus moderate exercise 4 to 6 days per week	1.7
Regular house chores plus strenuous exercise 3 to 4 days per week	1.8
Regular house chores plus strenuous exercise 4 to 6 days per week	1.9

Remember to subtract 250 to 500 calories from whatever BEE number you come up with in order to determine your daily calorie needs when trying to lose weight. Cutting back on this amount of calories leads to weight loss of ½ to 1 pound per week. That's a good thing because the more gradual the weight loss, the more likely it is that you're losing fat.

If you just want a simple, ballpark estimate, multiply your weight in pounds by the following numbers, depending on your activity level:

- ✔ If you're sedentary (little or no exercise), multiply by 10.

- ✔ If you're lightly active (exercising one to three days a week), multiply by 12.

- ✔ If you're moderately active (exercising three to five days per week), multiply by 15.

- ✔ If you're very active (exercising hard or playing a sport five to six days a week), multiply by 17.

- ✔ If you're extra active (exercising very hard or playing a sport six to seven days per week), multiply by 19.

As you age, you can boost your metabolism by continuing to be physically active and engaging in a strength-training program.

Eating from the Five Food Groups

 Before you begin tracking your eating habits, it's important to understand what you should be eating for optimal health. Most experts agree that eating a variety of foods from all five food groups is a great way to supply your body with the nutrients it needs. The five food groups include

- ✔ **Grains:** Foods that fall under the grains group are made from wheat, rice, oats, barley, cornmeal, or another cereal grain. So items such as breads, buns, crackers, cereal, pasta, rice, tortillas, and pita pockets are all considered grain products.

  Two categories of grains exist: whole grains and refined grains. Your goal is to include as many whole grains in your diet as possible. Making them at least half of your grain choices is preferable because whole grains provide more fiber and are generally more nutrient dense.

- ✔ **Fruits:** This category includes all types of fruits, whether fresh, canned, or frozen.

- ✔ **Vegetables:** Fresh, canned, and frozen veggies all belong in this group.

✔ **Meat and beans:** Members of this category include fish, poultry, beef, pork, eggs, dried beans, legumes, nuts, and soy products (think tofu).

✔ **Milk:** This group includes dairy products such as fluid milk, cheese, yogurt, and ice cream.

So where do potato chips and candy bars fit in? Well, they're considered extras — other foods that provide calories but in general don't provide many nutrients. These types of foods can fit into your diet, but you want to pay particular attention to the portion sizes of these foods.

Table 1-3 lists the nutrients each food group provides.

Table 1-3	Nutrients by Food Group
Grains	Fiber B vitamins (riboflavin, thiamin, niacin, folate) Minerals (iron, magnesium, selenium)
Fruits	Fiber Vitamins (vitamin C, folate) Minerals (potassium)
Vegetables	Fiber Vitamins (vitamins A, E, and C; folate) Minerals (potassium)
Meat and beans	Protein B vitamins (B6, niacin, thiamin, riboflavin) Vitamin E Iron Zinc Magnesium
Milk	Calcium Vitamin D Protein Potassium

For help visualizing the five food groups, head to www.mypyramid.gov, home of the United States Department of Agriculture's (USDA) MyPyramid, a visual tool that depicts the basic food groups and makes recommendations for proper choices for good health. The recommendations are based on the USDA's *Dietary Guidelines for Americans*.

Choosing snacks and planning meals around the five food groups is an easy approach to healthy eating. In particular, eating more fruits and vegetables may reduce your risk of stroke, cardiovascular disease, and diabetes.

What's a Serving?

When you keep a food journal, you absolutely have to be aware of how much you're eating. *A handful, a small spoonful,* and *some* aren't specific enough terms to really allow you to make progress in understanding how much food you're consuming. They also don't help you distinguish between a serving and a portion. A *serving* is the amount of food or drink designated by the manufacturer or the USDA guidelines; a *portion* refers to the amount of food or drink a person may consume.

In the next sections, we give you a better understanding of servings, from the daily recommendations for each food group to ideal serving sizes of popular foods, so you can better control your overall portion sizes. We also help you decipher the Nutrition Facts label and shine some light on the role beverages (including the alcoholic kind) play when you're counting calories.

The choices you make are important, but the portion sizes of the foods and beverages that you consume are perhaps more important. After all, eating healthfully isn't just about what you eat; it's also about how much you eat.

Serving size 101

Following are the basic daily serving recommendations for adults for each food group (we cover the five food groups earlier in this chapter):

- ✔ Grains: 5 to 11 servings
- ✔ Fruits: 2 cups
- ✔ Vegetables: 2 to 3 cups
- ✔ Meat and beans: 5 to 8 ounces
- ✔ Milk: 3 to 4 servings

Table 1-4 presents the serving sizes for popular food items by food group.

Table 1-4	Serving Sizes of Popular Foods
Grains	1 mini bagel 1 small biscuit 1 slice bread ½ English muffin ½ cup bulgur ½ cup barley 1 small piece cornbread 5 whole-wheat crackers 7 round crackers 1 small muffin 1 4-inch pancake ½ cup oatmeal or 1 packet instant 3 cups popcorn 1 cup flake-type, ready-to-eat cereal ½ cup rice ½ cup pasta 1 6-inch tortilla
Fruits	1 medium apple 1 large banana 1 large orange or peach About 8 strawberries 1 small wedge watermelon or 1 cup cubed
Vegetables	1 cup cooked greens or 2 cups raw About 12 baby carrots 1 large sweet potato 1 medium white potato 1 cup peas 1 cup corn 3 spears broccoli or 1 cup chopped 1 cup green beans 1 cup cucumber 2 cups lettuce
Meat and beans	1 ounce meat, poultry, or fish ¼ cup cooked dry beans 1 egg 1 tablespoon peanut butter ½ ounce nuts
Milk	1 cup milk or yogurt 1½ ounces hard cheese 2 ounces processed cheese

Every day, try to get about eight servings of grains, five serv-ings of fruits and vegetables, two servings (5 to 8 ounces total) of meat and/or beans, and three servings of dairy.

Thinking of serving and portion sizes in terms of everyday objects can help you visualize measurements that seem pretty darn vague otherwise. May we suggest the following visualiza-tion tricks?

✔ 1 teaspoon = A single die

✔ ¼ cup = An egg

✔ ½ cup = A tennis ball

✔ 3 ounces of meat, poultry, or fish = A deck of playing cards

✔ 2 ounces of cheese = 2 dice

✔ 1 cup of cereal, grain, fruits, or vegetables = A baseball

The Nutrition Facts label

The government-mandated Nutrition Facts label present on most packages of food in the United States is a valuable tool for determining how a food may fit into your personal dietary intake. As you can see in Figure 1-1, the Nutrition Facts label provides you with lots of information. For the purpose of weight loss, take a look at serving size, calories, fat, fiber, and sodium in particular.

When you pick up a package of food, first look at the serving size indicated on the Nutrition Facts label. This number helps you understand what a typical serving is for this particular food item. After you know the serving size, check out the listed calories. Keep in mind, though, that this number refers to the amount of calories for the serving size specified on the label.

As you review serving sizes, consider the portion you've doled out to yourself. If you're eating two servings' worth of an item, you must double the total calories and nutrients for that portion to have an accurate count of the calories and nutrients you're consuming.

Nutrition Facts

Serving Size 1/2 cup (75g)
Servings Per Container 6

Amount Per Serving

Calories 280   Calories from Fat 110

	% Daily Value*
Total Fat 12g	**18%**
Saturated Fat 1.5g	**9%**
Trans Fat 0g	
Polyunsaturated Fat 2g	
Cholesterol 0mg	**0%**
Sodium 20mg	**1%**
Total Carbohydrate 43g	**14%**
Dietary Fiber 10g	**38%**
Sugars 5g	
Protein 10g	

Vitamin A 0%	•	Vitamin C 0%
Calcium 6%	•	Iron 20%

*Percent Daily Values are based on a 2,000 calorie diet.

INGREDIENTS: Oat Bran, Rolled Oats, Barley, Rye, Sunflower Seed, Flax Seed, Chia Seed, Lecithin, Dried Apple, Apricots, Raisins, Walnuts, Almonds, Nutmeg, Vanilla

Figure 1-1: A sample Nutrition Facts label.

A note about beverages

The calories from beverages are often the calories people tend to forget about. After all, how can something with so little substance help you pack on pounds? Trust us when we say that a calorie is still a calorie. To have a solid understanding of the amount of calories you're consuming, you have to count the ones in your beverages.

Following is a rundown of the calories found in a 12-ounce serving of some common beverages:

- ✔ Cappuccino (lowfat), 109

- ✔ Chai (lowfat), 186

- ✔ Cranberry juice cocktail, 200

- ✔ Iced tea (sweetened), 100

- ✔ Lemonade, 180

  ✔ Orange juice, 150

  ✔ Regular soda, 150

  ✔ Sports drink, 95

Always be aware of the beverage portions you're ordering and consuming. A "small" drink is sometimes 16 ounces rather than 12 ounces. Watch out for those 20-ounce soda and juice bottles, too.

When keeping your journal, don't forget to record happy hours. Today's cocktail glasses have become supersized, and alcoholic beverages can add a *lot* of calories to your diet. Here's an approximate calorie guide for your favorite libations:

  ✔ 12-ounce beer, 150

  ✔ 12-ounce light beer, 100

  ✔ 5-ounce glass of white wine, 100

  ✔ 5-ounce glass of red wine, 120

  ✔ 7-ounce mixed drink (gin and tonic, rum and coke, and so on), 200

  ✔ 5-ounce sweet mixed drink (whiskey sour, daiquiri, and so on), 300

  ✔ 10-ounce margarita, 600

  ✔ 5-ounce vodka martini, 310

  ✔ 4-ounce cosmopolitan, 200

By becoming more aware of how many calories are in the beverages you drink, you may be motivated to add more water to your daily liquid intake. Not only is water good for you but it's also calorie free!

Chapter 2

Developing Goals You Can Stick With

*1*f you're like most people, you've set some ridiculous goals in your lifetime. You know the kind. They sound like this: "I'm never going to stay up that late again!" or "I'm giving up cookies for good!" Any goal that includes or implies the word *never* or *always* usually isn't going to be met with success. After all, you're only human.

Goals need to be realistic if you're ever going to achieve them. You also need to be motivated by an inner purpose in order to be successful in the long run. For example, losing 20 pounds as part of a team weight-loss challenge at work may not result in long-term success (that is, you may gain the weight back within six months) compared to setting individualized, short-term goals that result in personal weight loss and improved health markers (such as better blood pressure or lower cholesterol levels).

In this chapter, we help you create a vision and establish realistic, detailed goals so you can better use this journal as a tool for achieving success. We also get you thinking beyond the scale and looking at other ways of measuring your progress toward a healthier lifestyle.

Determining Which Stage of Behavior Change You're In

Behavior change is what makes weight loss and weight maintenance possible. The problem is that changing one's behaviors is difficult. Just think about this for a moment: If you're fairly physically healthy, you probably agree that taking a 20-minute walk five days a week and eating an apple a day is easy. But moving from thinking those things to actually *doing* them is another thing completely.

In order to bring about a real, lasting change in your behavior, you need to be aware of how truly committed you are to making a change. Enter the stages of behavior change. Developed by James Prochaska and his colleagues at the University of Rhode Island, the following stages of behavior change describe the process people go through in order to modify a problem behavior:

✔ **Pre-Contemplation:** When you're in this stage, you're not really recognizing a problem. People in this stage often make excuses to support their resistance to change.

✔ **Contemplation:** In this stage, you acknowledge the problem behavior and that you have a desire to change it, but you may not know how to begin. If you're stuck in this stage, ask yourself what's really preventing you from getting started.

Keeping a food and exercise journal can help you discover what's blocking you and how to get past it.

✔ **Preparation:** You're ready to make changes, and you understand the benefits of doing so. You're gearing yourself up mentally and working on a plan. Keeping a food and exercise journal at this stage helps you determine which behaviors to focus on.

Page one of your journal isn't going to be an outline of the perfect plan, but it *is* going to be a starting place from which you can grow.

When you're in the preparation stage, you may want to seek support. Consult your physician or a registered dietitian, or use some of the tools and support groups available online (we recommend Real Living Nutrition Services, found at www.reallivingnutrition.com, as a resource for reliable online nutrition coaching and information). You can also ask your family and friends to cheer you on along the way, but stick with the experts for advice.

✔ **Action:** In this stage, you're beginning to actively adjust the problem behavior. This is where you're putting your plan into motion, one goal at a time. Logging entries in this journal is an action step.

✔ **Maintenance:** The maintenance stage is where the problem behavior is stabilized. A person in this stage has lost weight, lowered cholesterol, or achieved better blood sugar control through changes in diet and exercise. At this stage, you must work on making your behavior changes permanent lifestyle changes. Keeping a journal can help you stay on track. You can also do it as a way to periodically "check in" with yourself.

Maintaining positive behavior changes allows you to reach your health goals.

✔ **Relapse:** Relapse occurs when you resort to old behaviors. When you experience a relapse, take a moment to identify what triggered it (perhaps it was a particular situation, like a vacation or a stressful time at work). Then build a support system so you're better equipped to face that trigger the next time it occurs.

By keeping a journal of what you eat and how often you exercise, you stand a better chance of overcoming relapses quickly so you can get back on the wagon toward better lifestyle choices.

In order to embark on behavior change, you must *decide* to change, which means you have to be ready to move quickly through the initial stages of behavior change and get to the action stage. This is often the missing link in the lose-weight-fast messages put out by the popular media. These information sources offer quick sound bites, but they don't support any particular behavior change that's necessary for success.

Creating a Vision

Your *vision* is what you're working toward. Before you start filling in the pages in Part III, you first need to take some time to really visualize what you want to achieve. Close your eyes and picture how you'll look and feel a year from now. Imagine how much stronger your body will be in two months after regular exercise. See yourself improving your race time. You get the idea.

Your vision is unique to you. Ask yourself why you want to make your vision a reality. Consider what that realized vision will bring to your life. Think about and write down a long-term vision and remember that successful weight loss isn't a short-term process but a lifelong one.

After you have a vision in mind, you can create a detailed, positive, action-oriented statement that explains it. Include what your vision is, why you're working on it, and how you're going to make it happen. Such a statement may sound something like this:

> *I'm going to lose 10 pounds so I can lower my cholesterol, manage my blood pressure, and feel better in my jeans. I plan to write weekly goals, complete a daily journal at least five days a week, and monitor my progress by checking off my goals and weighing myself weekly. I'll also get a report from my doctor at my annual exam to see whether I've lowered my cholesterol and kept my blood pressure in check.*

Using a food and exercise journal is a great way to get your vision out on paper and keep it in front of you as you work to meet your goals.

Setting SMART Goals

Stating a broad goal such as "I want to lose 20 pounds" doesn't give you any tools to use to actually begin losing weight. Also, such simple goals are often too lofty and can be discouraging when you don't get the results you want. The best goals are SMART, an acronym that stands for

- ✔ Specific
- ✔ Measurable
- ✔ Attainable
- ✔ Realistic
- ✔ Timely

We explain how to make your goals fit each of these characteristics in the next sections.

A quick word about motivation: Motivation is the activation of goal-oriented behavior. *Intrinsic motivation* comes from within; it's not fueled by outside reward or bribery. Goals like "I'm going to lose 10 pounds by using this food and exercise journal so I can feel better, live longer, and keep up with my active children" are a result of intrinsic motivation. *Extrinsic motivation* is dependent on outside influences. Goals like "my husband will buy me a diamond necklace if I lose 10 pounds" are based on extrinsic motivation. Motivation that comes from within promotes the most success toward fulfilling your goals.

Just because intrinsic motivation works better than the extrinsic kind doesn't mean you can't occasionally reward your positive behaviors and successes. Sometimes it's fun to add a little flair to your motivation. Feel free to "reward" yourself when you achieve a set of goals — just make sure the reward is a non-food-oriented treat. Some options include a new outfit, a fun day-trip, and a manicure or pedicure.

Specific goals

You have a greater chance of accomplishing a specific goal than a general goal. Specific goals help you understand what you need to do to work your way toward your ultimate goal. Table 2-1 shows just how easily you can turn general goals into more specific ones.

Table 2-1	General versus Specific Goals
General Goal	*Specific Goal*
I want to lose weight.	I plan to record my food and beverage intake in my journal daily.
I'll eat more fruit and snack less often.	I'm going to eat a piece of fruit daily at 10 a.m. and at 3 p.m., or in place of any other snack.
I'm going to exercise more.	I plan to meet my friend for a run on Monday, Wednesday, and Friday at 7:30 a.m.
I'll eat dinner in more often.	I'm going to plan and cook a simple dinner three nights a week.

To make your goals specific, follow this process:

1. **Ask yourself what you specifically want to accomplish.**

   Instead of saying "I want to get healthier," say, for example, "I want to lower my cholesterol so I stay healthy by reducing my risk of heart disease, and I want to lose weight so I can limit strain on my joints."

2. **Establish a time frame for achieving the goal.**

   Saying "I want to achieve my goals within the next year" is a good example.

3. **Identify any constraints that may hinder your progress and how you're going to conquer them.**

   For instance: "I'll plan around my work schedule by exercising at 6 a.m. or first thing in the morning before I shower, I'll limit baked goods in the house so I'm not tempted, and I'll set up a workout schedule to meet my friend at the gym so I won't skip it."

4. **Brainstorm reasons for accomplishing your goals.**

   Continuing with our example, you may come up with something like "I want to enjoy an active lifestyle by maintaining a healthy weight, and I want to feel more comfortable in my clothes and while performing daily activities."

Specific goals must be specific to you, not just specific in their wording. Your goals may not be the same as a friend's goals, even if you're working out together. You may both want to lose weight, but that doesn't mean you both have the same specific goals in mind. Your friend's goal may be to lose weight to stave off knee pain, whereas your goal may be to lose weight to reduce your blood pressure. Different people may set different short-term goals, even if the long-term goal is similar.

Take a few minutes each week to write a new specific goal in your journal. You can set up to three goals per week, but if you try to work on more than that, you may get overwhelmed. Working on a few realistic goals and allowing those behaviors to become habits before moving on to new goals is much better than working on tons of goals all at once and failing to achieve any of them.

Measurable goals

When you measure your progress toward a goal, you stay on track. Ask yourself questions such as the following to determine whether a particular goal is measurable:

- How much?
- How many?
- How will I know when it's accomplished?

Perhaps your goal involves cutting back on sugar. You can easily measure how much sugar you're cutting in terms of foods (such as sugary beverages, desserts, and doughnuts). For instance, you may have changed your daily morning doughnut behavior to eating only one doughnut on Fridays. You can easily track your goal to eat less sugar and your progress toward that goal in your journal.

Attainable goals

Goals become more attainable when you begin to make them specific and measurable. You can accomplish almost anything if you plan out the details and establish a time frame in which to accomplish them.

Setting a general goal, such as "I want to lose 20 pounds," becomes much easier when you frame it more specifically — think "I'll lose ½ to 1 pound a week" or "I'll lose 2 to 3 pounds a month." In the end, you'll lose 20 pounds over five to six months, which is both attainable and realistic.

Realistic goals

Any smart health or nutrition plan includes a set of realistic goals — in other words, goals that are actually doable. Realistic goals provide you with the tools you need and are built on the skills you have. If you love dessert, then setting a goal to never eat sweets probably isn't realistic. On the other hand, it may be realistic to limit dessert to just two days a week or to eat three servings of fruit daily before you reach for a sweet treat.

For your goals to be realistic, they must represent an objective that you're both willing and able to work on. Only you can decide what's doable for you. So for example, even though you may be willing to run a 5K race this coming weekend, you need to be able to admit that working toward running the next 5K race in a couple months may be a better idea considering you just started running last week.

A registered dietitian (RD) or certified health coach can help shed some light on whether a particular goal is realistic from a health perspective. For instance, even though you may think you can lose 20 pounds in one month, doing so is nearly physically impossible (or at least medically dangerous). An RD could tell you that trying to lose that much weight that quickly isn't safe or effective.

When setting your goals, you also want to consider your personal circumstances and history. If you're in your 20s, you may realistically be able to lose 10 pounds in ten weeks. If, however, you're in your 40s or 50s, it may be more realistic for you to lose 5 pounds in ten weeks. Consider your own reality when setting goals.

Although you want your goals to be realistic, this doesn't mean you shouldn't aim high. Often people have an easier time achieving more challenging goals than goals that are too easy because a low goal exerts low motivational force, whereas a higher goal can inspire you. Set the bar as high as you can!

Timely goals

Effective goals come with a time frame. Whether you aim to do something daily, weekly, or monthly, you need to define the time frame in which you plan to accomplish your goal. Why? Because putting an endpoint on a goal helps make it happen. Setting a deadline for the goal helps get you started and encourages you to dig right in. Following are some examples of what we mean:

- ✔ This week, I'll begin lifting weights two days a week for 45 minutes.

- ✔ I'll weigh myself every Wednesday to assess my progress.

> ✔ I'll lose 10 pounds in the next 12 weeks.
>
> ✔ I'll make an appointment with a personal trainer by the end of next week.

Don't be afraid to reevaluate. Say you set a time frame for weight loss over a four-month period, but at two months, you realize you aren't halfway toward your goal. That's okay. Set a new goal that's more attainable and realistic.

Thinking beyond the Scale

Achieving and maintaining a healthy body weight is a cornerstone to good health, which makes deciding to lose weight a worthy goal. However, losing weight is challenging, and maintaining weight loss is a lifelong commitment. Following are just some of the reasons why you may find losing weight to be a challenge:

✔ Perhaps you're a lifelong dieter, and your metabolism is therefore slower than it should be, making weight loss slower and more difficult.

✔ Maybe you're hitting middle age and finding that taking those 2 or 5 pounds off that you gained during vacation isn't as easy as it used to be.

✔ Perhaps you're an athlete who finds it difficult to fuel up and lose weight at the same time.

✔ Maybe you only need to lose 10 pounds, so weight loss is going slowly.

✔ Perhaps you've hit a weight-loss plateau and your body is clinging to that weight.

There's one similarity in all of these scenarios: The scale is playing far too important of a role.

Yes, weighing yourself is essential to evaluating your weight loss, but getting on the scale too often can be self-defeating. Weighing yourself every morning is okay if you're willing to accept the fact that it's normal for body weight to fluctuate from day to day, but in general, you only need to step on the scale once or twice a week. Why? Because no matter how much weight you want or need to lose, the number on the scale doesn't, and shouldn't, define you.

If you stay focused on the scale and you hit a weight-loss plateau, you may wind up feeling even worse about your progress — or lack thereof. A *weight-loss plateau* is when your body settles into a weight for a while even though you're continuing to eat well and exercise. Sometimes your body naturally overcomes such a plateau, and you begin losing weight again after a few weeks. Other times you may need to kick things up a notch by increasing the intensity of your exercise, adding different types of exercise, or reducing your calorie intake.

When you hit a weight-loss plateau, checking your weight daily or even weekly can be very discouraging. (And the mindset it puts you in can keep you stuck on that plateau.) If you're getting discouraged, take a break from the scale. Continue with your plan and your goals and then step back onto the scale in a week or two and see where you are.

You can successfully achieve your ideal weight and better health without dieting by

- ✔ Making a commitment to change your habits for the long term rather than focusing solely on losing weight

- ✔ Becoming educated about sound nutrition principles

- ✔ Logging your food and exercise in a journal

- ✔ Figuring out food-free ways to cope with emotions and stress

- ✔ Eating when you're hungry and stopping when you're full

- ✔ Shifting the focus from looking good to honoring your health and well-being

- ✔ Discovering how to adjust your food intake to match your activity level

- ✔ Forgiving yourself when you get off track (meaning if today didn't work out as well as you'd planned, let it go and move on to tomorrow)

- ✔ Seeking ongoing support to stay motivated

The best part about all of these activities is that they don't require you to obsess over the scale to track your progress. Take that, weight-loss plateaus!

Using Other Markers to Measure Success

Using a scale as the sole way of measuring your success can be frustrating (as noted in the preceding section). One of the best things about keeping a journal is that it not only helps you stay honest and on track but it also helps you evaluate the positive achievements you've made toward better health — achievements that have nothing to do with the scale.

Even if your ultimate goal is weight loss, take a good look at the positive things you're achieving. For instance:

✔ Have you made it to the gym three times a week?

✔ Are you able to lift more weight?

✔ Can you walk farther and faster?

✔ Did you trim minutes from your last race or triathlon?

✔ Are you eating more fruits and vegetables?

✔ Have you increased the fiber in your diet?

✔ Did your blood pressure come down?

✔ Did your LDL cholesterol level (the bad kind) drop?

✔ Did you lower your risk for diabetes or heart disease?

✔ Is your blood sugar under better control?

✔ Are you drinking more water?

✔ Are your jeans looser?

As you ask yourself these questions and others like them, you may be surprised to find that even though you haven't met your ultimate goal of losing weight, you've experienced all kinds of positive benefits from what you've accomplished thus far.

Fitness counts too. You may only be 4 pounds lighter than you were when you started strength training, but chances are you're much more fit because of your commitment to weekly physical activity. This is a winning situation! Muscle is denser than fat tissue, so you may indeed be losing some fat but also gaining some muscle.

Here are some other ways you can measure your success:

- ✔ **Compare the results of your blood work.** If you have high blood pressure, high cholesterol, or diabetes, consider phoning your doctor's office to find out what your past lab values were. Then make a note of your next appointment and track the changes in your blood pressure, HDL and LDL levels, or your overall diabetes management. If you do self-glucose monitoring at home, use that log along with this journal to see how your goals are working for you.

- ✔ **Use a pedometer to track your daily steps.** People who count their steps with a pedometer stay motivated to meet their exercise goals and lose weight. So why not consider making "I'm going to use a pedometer five days a week" one of your SMART goals? (We cover SMART goals earlier in this chapter.)

- ✔ **Turn your goals into a checklist for success.** So what if the scale is stuck for a while? Are you still setting and achieving goals (like successfully reducing portions and maintaining the right calorie intake)? If you continue to focus on setting SMART goals, you'll eventually begin to see results again; it may take some time, though, so be patient.

Chapter 3

Working toward Your Goals

● ●

In This Chapter

▶ Creating a new routine with the help of a food and exercise journal

▶ Discovering how many calories you burn in daily activities

▶ Picking up some exercise pointers and setting up an exercise schedule

● ●

*I*n Chapter 2, we show you how to set realistic goals so you can turn your bad habits into good ones. This chapter helps you determine how to go about accomplishing those goals with the help of a food and exercise journal, whether you want to lose weight, boost your fitness level, or improve certain health parameters (such as blood pressure, blood sugar, or cholesterol).

Creating a routine is an important part of forming a new habit. For instance, if one of your goals is to avoid the candy dish at work, you may try substituting a small bowl of mini pretzels or animal crackers at your desk. The same idea can apply to exercise goals. Energy in must be less than energy out for you to lose weight (see Chapter 1), so you have to figure out how to ensure the balance is right when it comes to your exercise plan. Perhaps all you need to do is establish a routine or exercise plan that really gets you moving. In this chapter, we help you figure out how to create a routine *and* an exercise plan so you have all the tools you need to achieve your goals.

How to Establish a Routine

A *habit* is a behavior pattern acquired by frequent repetition; a *routine* is a regular course of procedure. Creating a routine gives you a stronger chance of meeting your goals because it helps you develop daily habits. Slowly but surely, the new habits become an ordinary part of your daily life.

Before you can set a new routine filled with new, healthier habits, you need to figure out what your current routine is, complete with problem behaviors and any obstacles you face. In other words, you have to be aware of what's going on now. Do you have any idea whether you regularly skip meals, snack randomly, overeat at night, or skip your workouts? Keeping a food and exercise journal helps you recognize patterns in your behaviors so you can make positive changes to the choices that need improving.

Spend some time considering challenging situations you face and barriers to eating well and exercising. The following strategies can help you overcome some of these barriers:

- ✔ **Think.** It may sound simple, but trust us, it works. Think about the situations, places, and times when snacking or overeating is a challenge for you. Then plan ahead to deal with those situations.

- ✔ **Have healthy snacks around.** If you have plenty of healthy treats available, you'll eat healthier.

- ✔ **Remove your trigger foods.** *Trigger foods* are foods that automatically stir up thoughts such as "I can't stop eating these" or foods that lead to eating too much of other foods (like when you eat some chips and then want ice cream). Get rid of them.

- ✔ **Substitute another activity if you find yourself eating out of boredom.** Get up and take a ten-minute walk in the fresh air, climb some stairs in your building, or do whatever else will take your mind off of being bored.

- ✔ **Find a friend to exercise with or report to.** If you commit to someone else, you're more likely to get out there and exercise.

- ✔ **Commit to exercise.** You probably have more free time than you think. Why not commit to devoting some of it to exercise? Subscribe to a fitness magazine or e-newsletter; sign up for a weekly yoga, aerobics, spinning, or Zumba class; or pop in an exercise DVD or turn on a TV fitness program and work out at home.

✔ **Exercise in the morning.** People who schedule workouts in the morning are more likely to exercise consistently because there's less interference at this time of day.

✔ **Address medical issues.** You may have a health condition that's preventing you from eating better. Discuss any physical changes you've noticed with your doctor.

In general, eating on a regular schedule each day helps ensure you consume adequate nutrition and prevents you from becoming overly hungry. This is important because hunger control is one of the secrets to weight control.

No two people's schedules and responsibilities are alike. You may be a student, work days, work nights, work from a home office, or stay home and care for children. No matter what your schedule is like, it's important to establish a routine for eating and exercising. Here are our recommendations:

✔ Plan to eat about four to six times a day. Meals and snacks should incorporate the five food groups. (We list a person's daily requirements from the food groups in Chapter 1.)

✔ Don't allow more than three to four hours to pass between meals or snacks.

✔ Plan small, healthy snacks daily.

✔ Eat more of your calories during the part of the day when you're most active.

✔ Plan your exercise schedule (complete with specific days and times) into your calendar.

Logging Your Way to Success

People who struggle with weight often face many challenges and obstacles. Certain situations such as a medical condition or decreased metabolism may make losing weight tougher. (Society's increasing portion sizes, the availability of high-fat/high-calorie foods, and emotional eating don't help either.)

Whatever the specific reason(s), raising awareness about your habits and dealing with obstacles are essential to success. Enter the food and exercise journal.

Logging your dietary intake and physical activity gives you the knowledge you need to achieve your goals. Not only that, but if you journal for one month and then take a look at your weight change, we bet you'll be pleased with your progress. (After all, it takes about 21 to 30 days to break a habit.)

Whether you need to lose weight, gain better control of a health condition (such as diabetes), or improve your overall heart health (or all three!), maintaining a food and exercise journal can help keep you motivated and on track.

Cutting Calories, the Easier Way

Keeping your calorie consumption under control when you're trying to lose weight is one of those things that can be easier said than done, especially when you feel justified in filling up on pizza and beer at night because you were pretty active during the day. You can still enjoy those foods, but you need to think about how much you're eating and how often. In the case of the pizza and beer, one or two slices is enough pizza. Replace a third slice with a salad and swap water for one of the beers.

Follow these tips to control your calorie consumption:

- ✔ **Use less fat.** Ask for dressings, sauces, and gravies on the side when dining out. Use less margarine, butter, or cream cheese in general and opt for mustard rather than mayonnaise. Also, look for nonfat or lowfat dairy products, choose leaner cuts or types of meat, and pick fewer fried foods.

- ✔ **Add fiber.** Fiber helps you fill up faster, thereby reducing your overall calorie intake. So go ahead and eat more salads, beans, whole grains, and fresh fruit.

- ✔ **Have some protein with each meal or snack.** Protein helps you feel full, allowing you to eat less. Opt for lean choices such as an egg, lowfat cheese, baked or grilled fish or skinless poultry, and lowfat milk or yogurt.

✔ **Avoid mindless snacking.** Everyone eats mindlessly once in a while. Using this journal is the secret weapon to combat mindless munching. When you're writing down all of your food and beverage choices, you think twice about what and how much you're putting in your body.

✔ **Have healthy snacks around and plan them into your day.** Fresh fruit and raw vegetables are low in calories and loaded with important vitamins. Keeping some fruits washed and ready to eat and some veggies chopped and ready to grab or add to a sandwich plate makes healthy eating much easier.

✔ **Slow down.** Eating too quickly results in eating too much because you're not giving your brain enough time to cue your stomach that it's full. Taking sips of water between bites can help you slow down.

✔ **Use small plates and small packages.** Putting your food into a smaller bowl or onto a smaller plate helps trick your mind because portions look bigger in smaller containers. Opting for smaller packages also helps you control your portion sizes. For instance, if you're craving some candy-coated, chocolate-covered peanuts, don't go to the local big-box store and buy a case of 'em. Instead, buy one single-serving bag, enjoy it, and then be done with it.

✔ **Change the splurge routine.** Limit high-fat foods such as pizza and French fries to a once-a-week treat.

You aren't on a diet, but you *are* paying attention to what you eat in order to put your body on the road to better performance and health. Special foods or treats can still be part of your overall dietary intake — you just want to monitor the portion and frequency of them and, of course, write them down in your food and exercise journal.

Looking at the Calories Burned in Various Activities

Engaging in physical activity is an incredibly important part of adopting and maintaining a healthy lifestyle, but the concept can seem rather vague because people tend to think of physical activity strictly as "exercise." The truth is, every movement — whether you're vacuuming or jogging — counts in the long run because each one helps you burn calories.

Keeping track of the calories lost through each activity makes the concept of physical activity a much more tangible one in terms of weight loss.

Did you know that you can burn about 350 to 400 calories doing these common household chores?

- ✔ Washing and waxing a car for 45 to 60 minutes

- ✔ Washing windows or floors for 45 to 60 minutes

- ✔ Gardening for 30 to 45 minutes

- ✔ Pushing a stroller for 1.5 miles in 30 minutes

- ✔ Raking leaves for 30 minutes

- ✔ Shoveling snow for 15 minutes

- ✔ Walking up and down stairs for 15 minutes

Table 3-1 presents data from the President's Council on Fitness, Sports, and Nutrition and gets you acquainted with the calories burned while performing other various types of activities. The calorie estimates are broken down according to how strenuous the activity is, and the hourly estimates are all based on values calculated for calories burned per minute for a 150-pound person.

Table 3-1   Estimated Calories Burned by Activity

Type of Activity	Energy Costs in Calories per Hour
Sedentary	**Less than 150**
Lying down or sleeping	90
Sitting quietly	84
Sitting and writing, card playing, and so on	114
Moderate	**150–350**
Bicycling (5 mph)	174
Canoeing (2.5 mph)	174
Dancing (ballroom)	210
Golf (twosome, carrying clubs)	324
Horseback riding (sitting to trot)	246

Type of Activity	Energy Costs in Calories per Hour
Light housework, cleaning, and so on	246
Swimming (crawl, 20 yards/min.)	288
Tennis (recreational doubles)	312
Volleyball (recreational)	264
Walking (2 mph)	198
Vigorous	*More than 350*
Aerobic dancing	546
Basketball (recreational)	450
Bicycling (13 mph)	612
Circuit weight training	756
Cross-country skiing (5 mph)	690
Football (touch, vigorous)	498
Ice skating (9 mph)	384
Jogging (10-min. mile, 6 mph)	654
Racquetball	588
Roller skating (9 mph)	384
Scrubbing floors	440
Swimming (crawl, 45 yards/min.)	522
Tennis (recreational singles)	450

(Sources: "William D. McArdle, Frank I. Katch, Victor L. Katch, "Exercise Physiology: Energy, Nutrition and Human Performance" (2nd edition), Lea & Febiger, Philadelphia, 1986; Melvin H. Williams, "Nutrition for Fitness and Sport," William C. Brown Company Publishers, Dubuque, 1983.)

Running is a great way to burn calories. Walking is good too, but running generally gets you burning more calories faster, as you can see by working the formulas found in Table 3-2. Note that *total calorie burn* includes the energy your body uses even when you aren't exercising. The column related to *net calorie burn* measures calories burned, taking into account your basal metabolic rate, or BMR (flip to Chapter 1 to find out what yours is). ***Note:*** The walking formulas apply to speeds of 3 to 4 miles per hour; at 5 miles per hour and faster, walking burns more calories than running.

Table 3-2   Calories Burned While Running or Walking

Activity	Total Calorie Burn/Mile	Net Calorie Burn/Mile
Running	0.75 × Your weight (in lbs.)	0.63 × Your weight (in lbs.)
Walking	0.53 × Your weight (in lbs.)	0.30 × Your weight (in lbs.)

Adapted from "Energy Expenditure of Walking and Running," Medicine & Science in Sport & Exercise, Cameron et al, Dec. 2004.

Exercise alone isn't enough to make you lose weight, especially if you have the mentality that because you just burned, say, 250 calories walking, now you can eat a candy bar. To lose body fat, you have to look at the whole day's energy balance. If over the course of a day you create a calorie deficit by burning off more calories than you consume, you lose body fat. On the other hand, if you consume more calories than you burn, you gain body fat.

Exercise 101

A well-balanced exercise program includes cardiovascular (cardio) workouts and strength-training workouts. Cardio exercise (think jogging, walking, cycling, and swimming) helps exercise the heart muscle by raising the heart rate. It generally uses large muscle groups and requires more oxygen than strength training, a type of exercise that's important for building muscle mass (and includes weight lifting, yoga, and abdominal work). Because muscle tissue burns up more calories than fat tissue and you lose muscle quickly as you age, you want to stick with (or add) a strength-training component to your exercise program in order to maintain your muscle and metabolism.

Fitting exercise into your weekly schedule is vital. Ideally, you want to exercise a total of four or more days per week. Try to do three to four days of cardio and two to three days of strength training weekly (although you can do cardio and strength training on the same day if you prefer).

Choose activities that you enjoy doing, and you'll be more likely to keep them up. This is especially true if you're new to exercise. If, for example, swimming energizes you, start swimming laps or doing other water exercises at the local pool. The other thing you can do is just work on increasing your physical activity daily. No two people are at the same fitness level, and that's perfectly okay. Find what works for you and schedule it.

The following sections introduce you to some strength-training exercises you can try and present several workout plans to help you get moving.

 Always get your doctor's okay before beginning an exercise program.

Sampling some strength-training exercises

You don't have to go to a gym to do strength training, but a gym does offer a variety of equipment. Wherever you choose to do your strength training, here's an overview of the fun options that await you:

- ✔ **Weight lifting:** You can use either machines or free weights (dumbbells). Start with a weight that's difficult enough but that you're still comfortable with. You should be able to do one set of 8 to 12 repetitions with good form, with the last 2 repetitions feeling difficult. Increase your weights by 2½ to 5 pounds every week, making sure you can still do eight repetitions of each exercise.

- ✔ **Abdominal work:** This kind of exercise includes planks, ab crunches, and fitness ball work. If you prefer crunches, work up to three sets of 20 to 25 crunches per set.

- ✔ **Yoga or Pilates:** Yoga and Pilates build strength and balance. You can purchase a DVD to do at home, but it's best to start by taking some classes with a good instructor to get a foundation in the basics.

 If you don't do strength-training exercises properly, you may wind up hurting yourself. If you haven't exercised in a while, consider investing in a personal trainer who can set up a plan for you and show you proper form.

Planning your workouts

Coming up with a workout plan can be challenging, but doing so puts you one step closer to reaching your goals. We help you out by presenting some individual sample plans in this section. These sample workout plans are for you if you already include moderate exercise in your lifestyle and want to kick things up a notch. If you've never exercised but want to start, you can always modify these workouts to suit your needs.

If the sample workouts in this section seem out of your league, take heart and start slowly. At first, you may only be able to take a five-minute walk at a slow pace three times a day, but that's still great. Gradually keep at it, increasing your pace and total time until you can walk for 30 minutes daily. It may take you a month or more to build up to your goal, but doing so is well worth it. (For help setting goals, flip to Chapter 2.)

Table 3-3 features three sample exercise plans. Repeat one week's schedule for several weeks. If you find yourself growing bored or think the activities are getting easier, add time to the exercises or try different ones.

Table 3-3		Sample Weekly Exercise Plans				
SUN	*MON*	*TUES*	*WED*	*THURS*	*FRI*	*SAT*
Rest	Jog, 4 mi.	Lift weights, 45 min.	Walk, 3 mi.	Lift weights, 45 min.	Run intervals, 30 min.	Yoga class
SUN	*MON*	*TUES*	*WED*	*THURS*	*FRI*	*SAT*
Rest	Elliptical, 20 min.	Yoga DVD, 1 hour	Walk, 3 mi.	Weights DVD, 30 min.	Walk, 4 mi.	Walk, 2 mi.
SUN	*MON*	*TUES*	*WED*	*THURS*	*FRI*	*SAT*
Rest	Walk, 4 mi.	Lift weights, 45 min.	Walk, 3 mi.	Push-ups and abs, 15 min.	Rest	Bike, 15 mi.

Perhaps you have a treadmill that has been languishing in your garage or basement for months. What better time to break it back out than when you're trying to meet your week's goal of squeezing in more cardio exercise? Table 3-4 features a 60-minute interval treadmill workout designed to burn 500 calories. (An *interval* is one portion of a workout. Each interval changes pace throughout the workout, speeding up, then slowing down, and repeating. Interval workouts are great fat-burners.) The left-hand column of Table 3-4 tells you the interval, the middle column notes your pace, and the right-hand column tells you how long you need to keep that pace up (you can watch the minutes pass by on your treadmill clock).

Table 3-4   500-Calorie Treadmill Workout

Interval	Pace	Minutes
1	Jog, 5 mph	0:00–10:00 (warm up)
2	Sprint, 7.5 mph	10:01–10:20
3	Jog, 5 mph	10:21–11:20
4	Repeat intervals 2 & 3, twice	11:21–14:00
5	Jog, 5 mph	14:01–17:00
6	Run, 6.5 mph	17:01–27:00
7	Jog, 5 mph	27:01–31:00
8	Run, 6.5 mph	31:01–35:00
9	Jog, 5 mph	35:01–39:00
10	Repeat intervals 8 & 9, twice	39:01–55:00
11	Slow pace to a jog, then walk	55:01–60:00 (cool down)

Last but not least, Table 3-5 gives you a sample 30-minute workout you can perform on an elliptical. This machine has become a great alternative to the treadmill. It provides both a cardiovascular workout and a great leg and arm workout. The left-hand column in Table 3-5 tells you how many minutes to spend at the level noted in the right-hand column.

Table 3-5	200-Calorie Elliptical Workout
Minutes	*Level*
0–5	3 or 4 (warm up)
6–10	5 or 6
11–15	6 or 7
16–20	8 or 9
21–25	6 or 7
26–30	3 or 4 (cool down)

Part II
How to Use a Food and Exercise Journal

The 5th Wave   By Rich Tennant

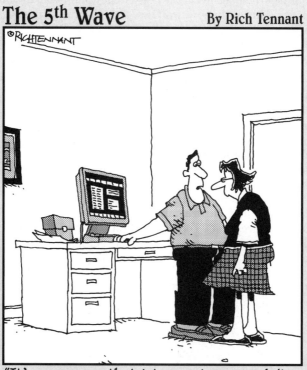

"It's a program that lets you log your daily caloric intake and then convert it to a crustless, lowfat pie chart."

In this part . . .

What's so hard about using a food and exercise journal? You just fill in the blanks, right? Yes and no. The secret to keeping a journal that helps you fulfill your health goals lies in the consistency and detail of your entries. This part shows you how to keep an effective log of your daily food and beverage intake as well as your physical activity. It also demonstrates how you can personalize the journal pages based on your health history and goals.

Even athletes can benefit by keeping a food and exercise journal because this tool isn't just for folks who want to lose weight and improve health. It's also for folks who want to enhance their physical performance. If you're an athlete, you know that the content and timing of your meals can really affect your performance. Logging your daily meal choices and physical activity therefore gives you the information you need to step up your game. That's why this part explains how to customize your journal and shares some sports nutrition basics and tips for achieving an optimal weight without sacrificing at the finish line.

Chapter 4

Dear Diary: Using Your Journal

- -

In This Chapter

▶ Familiarizing yourself with a food and exercise journal

▶ Writing detailed entries and personalizing your journal

▶ Discovering how to balance your dietary intake with physical activity

- -

*T*his chapter shows you, step by step, how to add detail to your journal so you can discover ways to improve or enhance your eating and exercise habits. We don't take a cookie-cutter approach to keeping a food and exercise journal, and you shouldn't either. You'll get the most out of your journal if you use it as a tool to help you personalize your eating and exercise plan. If you do, it'll help you achieve the specific health- and weight-related goals you've set for yourself (flip to Chapter 2 for guidance on setting goals).

Getting to Know Your New Best Friend: The Journal Layout

Taking a good look at the layout of this journal before you dive into it helps ensure you create meaningful daily entries. Also, understanding what you're going to be recording before you begin this process allows you to focus on your personal goals and not just random stuff. There's a page for each day of the week as well as a weekly assessment page to give you a better mental picture of how you did over the course of the week.

At the top of each daily page is a spot to write the date and your current weight. Note that if you record your weight each day, you're going to see some fluctuation (about ½ to 2 pounds) daily. You'll see progress over weeks or months, but if you don't think you can handle watching your weight go up and down each day, then skip this box. Or just weigh yourself once a week (like, say, every Tuesday) and write down your weight on that day.

Next up is a spot to write your goal for the day (which is actually just a reminder of your goal for the week, as we explain in the later "Being as Specific as You Can" section). Remember that you're not only setting goals for weight loss but also for making good food choices, improving your eating habits, and exercising. Don't just focus on the scale. (We help you figure out how to set realistic, attainable goals in Chapter 2.)

The following sections break down the remainder of what you can expect to find on each journal page and give you a visual of what we're talking about. They also explain how to use the weekly assessment page.

Your daily food and beverage journal

Each daily page of the journal includes a food and beverage section — space where you can track your food and drink, the times you eat or drink something, your mood (hungry, tired, bored, angry, upset, anxious, and so on), and your energy level.

Toward the top of each daily page are blank column headings. Feel free to fill these with the specific nutrients, calories, or points that you want to track and total those at the end of each day. We give you more details about how to personalize your journal later in this chapter. (For help determining how many calories or nutrients are in a food or beverage, look at the Nutrition Facts label on most packaged items or pick up a copy of *The Calorie Counter For Dummies,* written by us and published by Wiley.)

Last but not least is a section to track your water intake and fruit and vegetable intake. Both of these categories are important parts of a healthy, balanced diet. Consuming enough water (generally about six to eight glasses per day, depending on the amount of activity) and fruits and veggies (five or more servings daily) also aids in weight loss. Water not only helps you feel full and well hydrated but it also helps your body use the nutrients you consume. Fruits and veggies provide important nutrients, including vitamins A and C and *phytonutrients* (nutrients that are important to disease prevention). They also contain fiber, which helps control appetite.

Your daily exercise journal

The daily exercise section of the journal is where you track the type and duration of the exercises you do each day. If you want to, you can also enter the calories burned by performing each activity. Some pieces of exercise equipment (such as treadmills, elliptical machines, stationary bicycles, and rowing machines) tell you how many calories you burn during a workout. If, however, you want to give your mental muscles a workout too, you can use the information provided in Chapter 3 to figure out the calories you burn while performing different activities.

At the bottom of this section is a space for adding up the total number of minutes you exercised that day and the total amount of calories you burned. Work up to getting at least 30 to 60 minutes of exercise daily. As far as calories burned go, our motto is this: Some extra calories burned daily are better than no extra calories burned daily.

 Include all physical activity in your journal, even if you don't think of the activity as traditional exercise. Whenever you vacuum the house, do an hour of gardening, or walk from the farthest parking spot to your office, these activities (and more!) count toward living an active lifestyle.

A sample journal page

Words only go so far, which is why we want to take this opportunity to give you a preview of what a daily food and exercise journal page may look like with some entries filled in.

The sample journal page in Figure 4-1 shows you how you can make your entries. Note how specific the food and beverage entries are. This is the kind of detail you want in your journal. We delve into the importance of making your entries as specific as possible in the next section.

Day/Week	Date	Weight

Goals for the Day: _Drink more water_

Morning	Time: _7:30_	Cal			Mood	Energy
1 mini whole-wheat bagel		110			Rushed	Tired
1 TB light cream cheese		30				
8 oz nonfat milk		80				
	TOTAL	220				
Afternoon	Time: _12:30_					
Bowl vegetable soup		70			Hungry	Sleepy
Side salad w/ 2 TB Fr. dressing		90+80			Anxious	
16 oz water		0				
Medium apple		60				
	TOTAL	300				
Evening	Time: _6:30_					
Sloppy Joes (3 oz. meat, lg bun)		440			Hungry	Energized
Cole slaw, 1/2 cup		150				
16 oz water		0				
16 oz beer		150				
	TOTAL	740				
Snacks						
Honeydew, 4 sm pc Time: _10:30_		25				
String cheese, 1 pc Time: _3:30_		60				
12 oz coffee w/ 2 TB creamer Time: _3:30_		60				
1 oz pretzels Time: _7:30_		110				
	TOTAL	255				
Daily Totals		1,515				

Water/Fluid Intake
☑☑☑☑☐☐☐☐

Fruits/Vegetables
☑☑☑☑☐☐☐

Exercise Log

Type	Duration	Calories Burned
Run, 3.5 miles	35 min	
Weight lifting, upper body	45 min	
TOTAL	80 min	

Figure 4-1: A typical journal page with some entries filled in.

Your weekly assessment

Each weekly assessment page provides you with a spot to summarize your week. If you're a number-cruncher, you can write in each day's totals and then average them out. You can also enter how much exercise you did throughout the week. The goal is to wind up with an at-a-glance look at your overall dietary intake and exercise routine so you can set informed goals for the following week. Based on what you record, set goals for food choices, calorie intake, exercise, or any other lifestyle change you want to accomplish.

This portion of the journal is also intended to give you some positive reinforcement. After all, all this logging needs to pay off! Just when you think you aren't getting anywhere, take a moment to reflect on your accomplishments and then record them in the "Notes & Gold Star Moments" section of your weekly assessment page. So if you ate more vegetables, exercised for at least 20 minutes a day just like your goal stated you would, or consumed more high-calcium foods, record those moments and give yourself a well-deserved pat on the back.

Being as Specific as You Can

This journal is only going to be as good as the information you record in it. Consequently, the more specific your entries are, the better they'll serve you. At the very least, you should write a daily goal and track the specific food or beverage you consumed, how much you ate or drank (see Chapter 1 for the scoop on servings and portions), the time of day you ate, and whatever physical activity you engaged in that day.

We focus on encouraging behavior change, but if you aren't seeing weight loss after making several changes, or if you have a minimal amount of weight to lose, we recommend also tracking your calories as part of your minimum daily journal entry. After a few months pass and you have a better idea of the calories you're consuming, you may not have to worry about them so much.

When you record your food and beverage intake, try to include as much detail as possible. It's the specific detail that helps you figure out where you need to tweak things. For instance, you may look back over your day or week and notice that you're snacking out of control at 4 p.m. At next glance, you see that you aren't eating enough at lunchtime. Thanks to this knowledge, you can fix the afternoon snack binge by adding a serving of fruits, vegetables, or grains to your lunch-time meal to hold you over and control your afternoon snack portion.

Table 4-1 gives you an idea of the kinds of entries that are helpful and those that are pretty much worthless.

Table 4-1	How to Write Specific Entries
Write This	*Not That*
1 cup wheat squares, 4 oz 1% milk	Cereal and milk
2 slices whole-wheat bread, 3 oz turkey breast, lettuce, tomato, 1 tsp mustard; 1 oz bag potato chips; 1 medium apple	Sandwich, chips, apple
16 oz water	Water
8 wheat crackers, 2 oz cheddar cheese	Some cheese and crackers
1 large fried chicken breast, ½ cup mashed potatoes, 1 tsp butter	Chicken with potatoes
½ cup microwaved green beans, no butter	Green beans
12 oz light beer	Beer

Using measuring cups and spoons can be very eye-opening. If you eat cereal in the morning, for example, use the bowl you usually do and pour the dry cereal into a 1-cup measuring cup. (Why 1 cup? Because that's a common serving size for cereal. Check the label on your favorite cereal box and compare to see whether the serving size for that product differs.) Take a good look at how that 1 cup lands in your cereal bowl so you know how high to fill the bowl tomorrow. For foods that fall into the fat category (think peanut butter, cream cheese, salad dressing, or mayonnaise), use a tablespoon. Test out how much you're using of XYZ and compare it to the tablespoon. Then read the Nutrition Facts label on the product packaging to determine how many calories or how much fat is in a 1-tablespoon portion so you can record the information in your journal.

Don't forget to track your snacks! Snack portions can get out of hand quickly, especially if you eat your snacks out of the container they come in. Don't write "a handful of nuts" in your journal until you figure out how big your handful is. Nuts, for example, are a great snack and very nutritious, but they're also quite high in calories. Measure out ¼ cup of your favorite nut mix and then try to stick with that portion for your snack (there are 160 to 175 calories in ¼ cup of most nuts).

Of course, being specific doesn't just apply to your journal entries. It also applies to your goals. Creating a weekly goal helps you target any problem areas in your eating and exercise plan, and writing out that goal daily helps reinforce your overall vision (we help you develop your vision in Chapter 2). Adding detail to your goals improves your chances of achieving them.

Making It Personal

Using this journal for weight loss is a great idea, but there are other ways to make it a helpful tool for you. For example, if you have a history of, say, high cholesterol, high blood pressure, or diabetes, you can customize the daily journal pages to track some values that are particular to your personal situation. Specifically, you can customize the blank column headings on the daily journal pages to track whatever you want.

Following are a few ways to personalize your journal:

> ✔ **If you have high cholesterol:** You may want to include a column for tracking saturated fat (abbreviated Sfat) to remind yourself to read labels and log in the exact amounts. You may also want to create a Fiber column heading because a high-fiber diet (especially the soluble fiber found in foods such as oats, apples, dried beans, and bran) helps lower cholesterol.

Most women should limit their saturated fat intake to about 14 to 16 grams per day; men should limit theirs to 17 to 20 grams daily. (Total fat should be 30 percent of total calories, which is about 60 to 70 grams a day for most adults.) Optimal fiber intake is about 24 grams per day. However, if you don't already eat a lot of fiber, you should add it to your diet gradually — otherwise, you'll experience some serious discomfort. When pumping up your fiber intake, be sure to drink plenty of water to help avoid constipation.

✓ **If you have diabetes:** You may want to include your blood sugar readings and carbohydrates consumed in your daily journal pages. Looking at blood sugar levels through the day, along with your calorie intake and exercise, can help you achieve better blood glucose control.

Taking this information to your physician or diabetes educator can help her advise you about your overall blood glucose control and meal plan.

✓ **If you have high blood pressure:** Too much sodium can send blood pressure soaring, so you may want to create a Sodium column heading (abbreviated Sod). In addition to eating a moderate amount of sodium, you want to either lose weight or maintain a healthy weight (that's a BMI between approximately 19 and 24; see Chapter 1 for the scoop on BMI), eat plenty of fruits and vegetables (at least eight servings), and get enough lowfat dairy in your diet. Using the check boxes for fruit and veggie intake at the bottom of each daily journal page can help you meet your goal, and setting a goal to "include three servings of lowfat dairy products daily" can help you lower blood pressure.

✓ **If you just want to lose weight:** You may be able to get by with just logging the food or beverage, the exact portion, and calories in order to get a better handle on your overall dietary intake and eating patterns (if you already eat healthy foods, that is). However, paying attention to your mood, energy level, and how you eat (too fast, larger portions, or while you're doing something else) is also important. Tracking this information can help you figure out why you're eating at times when you may not be hungry.

Figure 4-2 shows you how a person with diabetes may customize her daily journal pages to track saturated fat (because diabetes increases one's risk for heart disease), carbohydrates, and fiber (in addition to calories).

Morning	Time:___:___	Sfat	Carb	Fiber	Cal	Mood	Energy
	TOTAL						

Figure 4-2: Customize your journal headings to track what you want.

Balancing Healthy Eating with Exercise

No matter how healthy your diet becomes, you're not truly living a healthy lifestyle until you start incorporating some element of exercise. Exercise improves cardiovascular health and your overall fitness level. Being fit allows you to do more, remain strong and flexible, and have better balance as you age.

Despite the claims of many weight-loss ads, there are no magic bullets when it comes to weight loss. To maintain your weight, you have to consume the proper amount of calories (that is, the amount of calories your body needs for the activities that you do; see Chapter 1). In other words, calories in must equal calories out to keep your weight consistent.

To lose weight, you must create a calorie deficit by either eating less or exercising more. To lose 1 pound a week, you have to create a calorie deficit of 500 calories per day. To do this, you must either cut back on your calorie intake or use more energy by exercising. So you could, for instance, eat 250 calories less and walk for 45 minutes, burning about 250 calories in the process, for a total calorie deficit of 500.

Get as much exercise as you can, with your physician's approval. The President's Council on Fitness, Sports, and Nutrition recommends that adults get 30 minutes of activity at least five days per week. (Children should get 60 minutes of activity daily.)

Chapter 5

A Special Message for Athletes

*W*hether you're an elite athlete, a recreational athlete, or a gym rat, eating affects your performance. In fact, physical activity, athletic performance, and recovery from exercise are all enhanced by optimal nutrition. And that's not just our opinion — it's the official position of the American Dietetic Association, the Dietitians of Canada, and the American College of Sports Medicine.

In this chapter, we help you better understand basic sports nutrition, show you how tracking your dietary intake and physical activity helps you perform better in the long run, and explain why you should opt for eating well and developing an effective training schedule instead of relying on expensive supplements to give you an edge. And because even athletes sometimes need to lose weight to compete, we also include guidelines for weight loss.

The Basics of Sports Nutrition

Everyone, athlete or not, needs different amounts of energy (in the form of calories), nutrients, and fluids. Athletes however, need to pay close attention to the specifics. How much, when, and what you eat affects how your body performs, so if you want it to perform well on demand, you need to keep several points in mind:

✔ **Consume adequate calories to support high-intensity training and maintain a healthy body weight.** We help you figure out how many calories you need to consume based on your activity level in Chapter 1.

✔ **Monitor your performance or progress toward goals based on your improved speed, strength, and endurance, not just your body weight or composition.** Optimal body fat depends on your gender, age, genes, and sport. Consequently, you may just be naturally inclined to weigh a little more or be less shapely than your fellow competitors. Focusing on other performance parameters helps you see progress beyond your body weight and natural body shape.

✔ **If you need to lose weight, work on this during the off-season or after a big competition (like a race).** You don't want to sacrifice performance when you're "in season," but that's exactly what happens if you restrict your calories too much during this time. We offer tips for losing weight as an athlete later in this chapter (for general calorie-cutting tips, flip to Chapter 3).

The next sections offer insight into how to keep your body properly fueled throughout the day.

Before exercising

Providing your body with fuel is a good idea before competing or exercising. However, there are no magic meals or snacks that can give you the cutting edge. What you eat on a day-to-day basis is what's really important, which is why you want to build a good nutrition base.

All the standard principles of balanced nutrition apply for athletes (we cover these in Chapter 1), but as an athlete, you should be aware of some additional nutritional pointers:

✔ **Carbohydrates provide energy, maintain blood sugar levels during exercise, and replace muscle *glycogen* (the storage form of carbohydrate).** The amount of carbohydrate you need depends on your sport and daily calorie needs, but in general, athletes should consume 2.7 to 4.5 grams of carbohydrate per pound of body weight.

If you're an endurance athlete, carbohydrates are your primary fuel source. According to the American College of Sports Medicine, 50 to 60 percent of energy used during one to four hours of continuous exercise is carbohydrate; the rest is from fatty acid oxidation. Training doesn't alter the amount of calories you burn, but it does alter the ratio of carbohydrate to fat burned. Therefore, the more fit you are, the better your body burns up fat for energy.

✔ **Protein provides energy and helps athletes maintain and repair muscle.** If you participate in endurance sports or do regular strength training, your daily protein intake should range from 0.5 to 0.8 grams per pound of body weight. You can easily get this amount of protein from your diet alone, without the use of protein or amino acid supplements. Foods in the meat/bean and dairy groups are primary protein sources; turn to Chapter 1 for the full scoop on the food groups.

✔ **Fat is an important source of energy that supplies some fat-soluble vitamins and provides essential fatty acids.** Try to get 20 to 35 percent of your daily calorie intake from fat.

✔ **Hydration is essential for everyone but for athletes in particular.** Dehydration decreases exercise performance, so adequate fluid intake before, during, and after exercise is important. Your goal should be to drink enough water to prevent dehydration. Sports drinks have their place (they provide a bit of carbohydrate, electrolytes, and fluid), but water is crucial.

Before training or competing, have a snack or meal that's relatively low in fat and provides carbohydrate for energy and some protein. Try to eat this meal or snack about two to four hours before you get moving (depending on your tolerance for eating before engaging in your sport). Of course, you should also make sure the food is something you enjoy eating. Don't forget to hydrate yourself too. Down an 8- to 16-ounce glass of water with your preworkout meal and then sip water up until your competition if you have to wait around.

While exercising

Keeping yourself hydrated during any type of exercise or competition is beneficial for replacing lost fluid. This is where a sports drink can come in handy. Sports drinks replace fluid as well as electrolytes (such as sodium and potassium) that the body loses when it sweats.

For endurance sports, such as long-distance cycling, triathlons, marathons, and any other event that lasts more than an hour, the primary goal is to provide the body with enough carbohydrate to replenish energy levels. Endurance athletes often use special nutrition products such as sports gels (a packaged, gooey, thick liquid providing easy-to-ingest pure carbohydrate in the form of sugar), sports nutrition bars (chewy, cookielike bars that provide carbohydrate and protein in an easy-to-carry package), and even sports beans (jelly beans with added sodium and potassium) for a quick energy boost. But not all athletes use these products. Some prefer to rely on bananas or fruit-filled cookies for carbohydrate because these foods are inexpensive, easy to carry, and easy to eat and digest.

After exercising

You should consume about 200 to 350 calories or so after a workout, making sure those calories are a combination of carbohydrate and protein. The carbohydrate helps restock your body's energy stores, and the protein helps your body build and repair muscle tissue. (You need about 0.5 to 0.7 grams of carbohydrate per pound of body weight within 30 minutes of exercising; after that, every two hours for four to six hours after exercise is adequate.)

After engaging in strenuous exercise, you should drink 16 to 24 ounces of fluids for every pound of body weight you lost through sweat. You can determine how much fluid you lost by first checking your weight in the morning or before your event and then weighing yourself again afterward. *Note:* If you go the sports drink route in order to replenish your carbs and electrolytes at the same time, drink just 8 to 12 ounces of fluid and remember to sip on water throughout the day as well.

Here are some quick postevent recovery snacks that provide about 10 to 20 grams of protein and 45 to 65 grams of carbohydrate:

✔ Sixteen ounces of lowfat chocolate milk

✔ A sports bar and an 8-ounce glass of lowfat white milk

✔ An 8-ounce fruit yogurt and a banana

✔ Two ounces of cheese with ten crackers plus an 8-ounce glass of 100-percent fruit juice

Logging Your Way to Better Performance

Taking the time to ensure that you're well fed and well hydrated is worth the effort, and keeping a food and exercise journal can help you develop an eating plan and stick to it.

If you're an endurance athlete, you're probably already familiar with journaling. Perhaps you enjoy logging your mileage, average speeds and times, and personal bests. If so, then you know all about the motivation and information you get from logging those things. Writing down what you eat can help you determine whether your performance (good or bad) is linked to your eating habits. It can also help you out if you need to shed a few pounds.

Note: Although endurance athletes often feel the immediate negative effects of improper eating, proper nutrition is important even if you're into nonendurance sports. If you play basketball, football, baseball, volleyball, golf, tennis, lacrosse, or anything else, you can also benefit from eating well and planning ahead.

As you customize the journal pages in Part III:

✔ Include a daily or weekly goal that relates to both your eating habits and your sport performance.

✔ Record your fluid intake. Note that you may need to drink additional fluids when you're active, especially in warmer weather.

✔ Track carbohydrate and protein in addition to calories.

✔ Manage your workout schedule.

✔ Use the weekly assessment page to record notes about your body measurements (waist, hips, thighs, and arms) to determine whether you're losing inches. This loss may or may not show up on the scale as you lose body fat, but it's still a good indication of weight loss and health, and it can have a positive effect on your performance.

Supplements: Too Much of a Good Thing

The sports nutrition industry is a billion-dollar business, and the increased number and availability of nutritional supplements is astounding — and mostly unregulated. All supplement manufacturers are required by the United States Food and Drug Administration to analyze the identity, purity, and strength of their products' ingredients, but they aren't required to demonstrate the safety and efficacy of their products.

Although some *ergogenic aids* (in this case, a nutritional or pharmaceutical supplement that enhances physical performance) may be helpful for athletes (for instance, glucosamine and chondroitin sulfate have been shown to help with joint lubrication), most are unnecessary. We don't recommend supplements as ergogenic aids for two reasons:

✔ Very few have been proven to improve performance.

✔ Some are unsafe.

You can achieve better fitness and performance without resorting to nutritional supplements by eating well and training smart. (See Chapter 1 for tips on how to build a good nutrition base.) Popping a pill doesn't help if you don't do the work. Nothing can replace effective training.

If you want to find out about safe supplementation or if you need help figuring out how to eat and train better, set up a meeting with a *sports dietitian* (a registered dietitian who specializes in sports nutrition). He can provide you with a complete nutrition assessment, help you select foods and create meal plans, and aid you in deciphering the myriad of sports nutrition choices so you can achieve your body's peak performance. A sports dietitian can also help you track your outcomes, address energy balance issues, and clear up any nutrition misinformation you may have previously encountered.

How to Lose Weight and Compete

Staying at an optimal weight for your height and body type improves your overall athletic performance, but if you find yourself carrying around a few extra pounds, losing that body fat may have more of an effect on your performance than making particular food choices. Don't get us wrong. Healthy eating helps support performance, but if you've been toting around an extra 10 pounds, you'll also see improvements in performance after reaching a healthier weight.

 If you're training for your first big competition (like a triathlon) next month, now isn't the time to start losing weight. Focus on that after the event. (We explain why you shouldn't try to lose weight before a big athletic competition or during a sports season in the earlier "The Basics of Sports Nutrition" section.)

Some athletes may have trouble balancing their dietary intake with their training and competition. We know you're working out or training regularly, but if you need to drop a few pounds to reach a more optimal weight, give some of the following suggestions a shot:

- ✔ **Assess your body fat.** Figuring out your body mass index (BMI) is your best bet for determining how much body fat you have; we tell you how to do just that in Chapter 1. Note, though, that as an athlete, you may be carrying more lean tissue (muscle) than fat, so you may weigh more than a non-athlete friend.

- ✔ **Steer clear of fad diets.** These diets don't work, plain and simple. Instead of following one, use this journal to help you set goals, get specific about eating behaviors that have been barriers to your weight loss in the past, and gradually lose weight (no more than 1 pound per week).

✔ **Keep balance and moderation in mind.** Honestly, most foods are okay as long as you don't overdo it. On the flip side, don't completely deprive yourself or limit or eliminate entire food groups.

✔ **Create a calorie deficit.** To lose 1 pound per week, you need to create a 500-calorie deficit each day. A good way to do this is by reducing your calorie intake while boosting your physical activity (either the level of intensity or what you do).

✔ **Fuel your workouts.** Consuming fewer calories doesn't mean skipping meals or snacks. While you're creating a calorie deficit, don't restrict the wrong foods at the wrong times. Be sure to eat before your workouts, don't skip meals, and plan healthy snacks.

✔ **Make sure you're eating enough carbohydrates.** Athletes require more energy than non-athletes, and people get their energy from carbohydrates. Athletes therefore need carbs. Your goal can be to manage your carbohydrate intake, but you shouldn't try to eliminate carbs from your diet.

✔ **Recover properly from exercise.** Don't deprive yourself of food after a workout. If you don't have that small snack afterward to replace your body's energy stores, you may *bonk* (lose all of your energy) during your next workout. Recovering properly also means consuming enough fluids. See the earlier "After exercising" section for an idea of how much to drink.

Part III
Journal

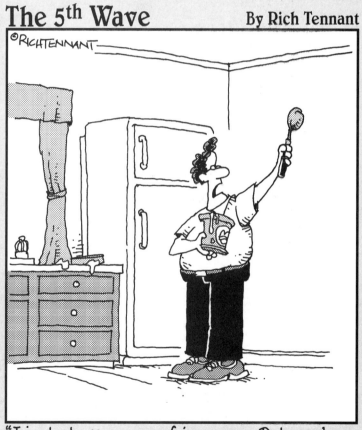

"I just ate 12 scoops of ice cream. Put me down for a dozen reps!"

In this part . . .

This part is where the magic happens. Following are 24 weeks' worth of blank journal pages that you can customize to fit your needs, as well as weekly assessment pages so you can see your weekly information at a glance, note your accomplishments, and set goals for the upcoming week.

Okay, so keeping a food and exercise journal isn't technically magic, but research has shown that people who record their food intake are more successful at losing weight and keeping it off than those who don't keep a journal. So start logging, dear reader! We're confident that after filling up all of these pages, you'll have healthier habits that will last you a lifetime.

Day/Week	Date	Weight	**67**

Goals for the Day: _____

Morning	Time: __ __:__ __					Mood	Energy
TOTAL							
Afternoon	Time: __ __:__ __						
TOTAL							
Evening	Time: __ __:__ __						
TOTAL							
Snacks							
	Time: __ __:__ __						
	Time: __ __:__ __						
	Time: __ __:__ __						
	Time: __ __:__ __						
TOTAL							
Daily Totals							

Water/Fluid Intake
❏ ❏ ❏ ❏ ❏ ❏ ❏ ❏

Fruits/Vegetables
❏ ❏ ❏ ❏ ❏ ❏ ❏ ❏

Exercise Log

Type	Duration	Calories Burned
TOTAL		

68

Day/Week	Date	Weight

Goals for the Day: _____

Morning Time: __ __:__ __					Mood	Energy
TOTAL						
Afternoon Time: __ __:__ __						
TOTAL						
Evening Time: __ __:__ __						
TOTAL						
Snacks						
Time: __ __:__ __						
Time: __ __:__ __						
Time: __ __:__ __						
Time: __ __:__ __						
TOTAL						
Daily Totals						

Water/Fluid Intake
❑ ❑ ❑ ❑ ❑ ❑ ❑ ❑

Fruits/Vegetables
❑ ❑ ❑ ❑ ❑ ❑ ❑ ❑

Exercise Log

Type	Duration	Calories Burned
TOTAL		

Day/Week	Date	Weight	**69**

Goals for the Day: _____

Morning Time: __ __:__ __					Mood	Energy
TOTAL						
Afternoon Time: __ __:__ __						
TOTAL						
Evening Time: __ __:__ __						
TOTAL						
Snacks						
Time: __ __:__ __						
Time: __ __:__ __						
Time: __ __:__ __						
Time: __ __:__ __						
TOTAL						
Daily Totals						

Water/Fluid Intake
❑ ❑ ❑ ❑ ❑ ❑ ❑ ❑

Fruits/Vegetables
❑ ❑ ❑ ❑ ❑ ❑ ❑ ❑

Exercise Log

Type	Duration	Calories Burned
TOTAL		

70

Day/Week	Date	Weight

Goals for the Day: _____

Morning Time: __ __:__ __					Mood	Energy
TOTAL						
Afternoon Time: __ __:__ __						
TOTAL						
Evening Time: __ __:__ __						
TOTAL						
Snacks						
Time: __ __:__ __						
Time: __ __:__ __						
Time: __ __:__ __						
Time: __ __:__ __						
TOTAL						
Daily Totals						

Water/Fluid Intake
☐ ☐ ☐ ☐ ☐ ☐ ☐ ☐

Fruits/Vegetables
☐ ☐ ☐ ☐ ☐ ☐ ☐ ☐

Exercise Log

Type	Duration	Calories Burned
TOTAL		

Day/Week	Date	Weight

Goals for the Day: _____

Morning	Time: __ __:__ __					Mood	Energy
TOTAL							
Afternoon	Time: __ __:__ __						
TOTAL							
Evening	Time: __ __:__ __						
TOTAL							
Snacks							
	Time: __ __:__ __						
	Time: __ __:__ __						
	Time: __ __:__ __						
	Time: __ __:__ __						
TOTAL							
Daily Totals							

Water/Fluid Intake
☐ ☐ ☐ ☐ ☐ ☐ ☐ ☐

Fruits/Vegetables
☐ ☐ ☐ ☐ ☐ ☐ ☐ ☐

Exercise Log

Type	Duration	Calories Burned
TOTAL		

72

Day/Week	Date	Weight

Goals for the Day: _____

Morning Time: __ __:__ __					Mood	Energy
TOTAL						
Afternoon Time: __ __:__ __						
TOTAL						
Evening Time: __ __:__ __						
TOTAL						
Snacks						
Time: __ __:__ __						
Time: __ __:__ __						
Time: __ __:__ __						
Time: __ __:__ __						
TOTAL						
Daily Totals						

Water/Fluid Intake
☐ ☐ ☐ ☐ ☐ ☐ ☐ ☐

Fruits/Vegetables
☐ ☐ ☐ ☐ ☐ ☐ ☐ ☐

Exercise Log

Type	Duration	Calories Burned
TOTAL		

Day/Week	Date	Weight	**73**

Goals for the Day: _____

Morning	Time: __ __:__ __						Mood	Energy
TOTAL								

Afternoon	Time: __ __:__ __							
TOTAL								

Evening	Time: __ __:__ __							
TOTAL								

Snacks								
	Time: __ __:__ __							
	Time: __ __:__ __							
	Time: __ __:__ __							
	Time: __ __:__ __							
TOTAL								
Daily Totals								

Water/Fluid Intake
☐ ☐ ☐ ☐ ☐ ☐ ☐ ☐

Fruits/Vegetables
☐ ☐ ☐ ☐ ☐ ☐ ☐ ☐

Exercise Log

Type	Duration	Calories Burned
TOTAL		

Food Intake Summary

DAY 1				
DAY 2				
DAY 3				
DAY 4				
DAY 5				
DAY 6				
DAY 7				
Weekly Total				
Average Daily Intake (Total ÷ 7)				

Did you meet your goals for water and fruit and veggie intake this week?   Yes   No

Exercise Summary

	Type	Duration	Calories Burned
DAY 1			
DAY 2			
DAY 3			
DAY 4			
DAY 5			
DAY 6			
DAY 7			
TOTALS			

Notes & Gold Star Moments

Goals for Next Week

Eating:

Exercise:

Other:

Day/Week	Date	Weight	75

Goals for the Day: _____

Morning	Time: __ __:__ __					Mood	Energy
TOTAL							
Afternoon	Time: __ __:__ __						
TOTAL							
Evening	Time: __ __:__ __						
TOTAL							
Snacks							
	Time: __ __:__ __						
	Time: __ __:__ __						
	Time: __ __:__ __						
	Time: __ __:__ __						
TOTAL							
Daily Totals							

Water/Fluid Intake
☐ ☐ ☐ ☐ ☐ ☐ ☐ ☐

Fruits/Vegetables
☐ ☐ ☐ ☐ ☐ ☐ ☐ ☐

Exercise Log

Type	Duration	Calories Burned
TOTAL		

76

Day/Week	Date	Weight

Goals for the Day: _____

Morning Time: __ __:__ __					Mood	Energy
TOTAL						
Afternoon Time: __ __:__ __						
TOTAL						
Evening Time: __ __:__ __						
TOTAL						
Snacks						
Time: __ __:__ __						
Time: __ __:__ __						
Time: __ __:__ __						
Time: __ __:__ __						
TOTAL						
Daily Totals						

Water/Fluid Intake
☐ ☐ ☐ ☐ ☐ ☐ ☐ ☐

Fruits/Vegetables
☐ ☐ ☐ ☐ ☐ ☐ ☐ ☐

Exercise Log

Type	Duration	Calories Burned
TOTAL		

Goals for the Day: _____

Morning	Time: __ __:__ __						Mood	Energy
TOTAL								
Afternoon	Time: __ __:__ __							
TOTAL								
Evening	Time: __ __:__ __							
TOTAL								
Snacks								
	Time: __ __:__ __							
	Time: __ __:__ __							
	Time: __ __:__ __							
	Time: __ __:__ __							
TOTAL								
Daily Totals								

Water/Fluid Intake
❑ ❑ ❑ ❑ ❑ ❑ ❑ ❑

Fruits/Vegetables
❑ ❑ ❑ ❑ ❑ ❑ ❑ ❑

Exercise Log

Type	Duration	Calories Burned
TOTAL		

78

Day/Week	Date	Weight

Goals for the Day: _____

Morning	Time: __ __:__ __					Mood	Energy
TOTAL							
Afternoon	Time: __ __:__ __						
TOTAL							
Evening	Time: __ __:__ __						
TOTAL							
Snacks							
	Time: __ __:__ __						
	Time: __ __:__ __						
	Time: __ __:__ __						
	Time: __ __:__ __						
TOTAL							
Daily Totals							

Water/Fluid Intake
❑ ❑ ❑ ❑ ❑ ❑ ❑ ❑

Fruits/Vegetables
❑ ❑ ❑ ❑ ❑ ❑ ❑ ❑

Exercise Log

Type	Duration	Calories Burned
TOTAL		

Day/Week	Date	Weight	**79**

Goals for the Day: _____

Morning	Time: __ __:__ __					Mood	Energy
TOTAL							
Afternoon	Time: __ __:__ __						
TOTAL							
Evening	Time: __ __:__ __						
TOTAL							
Snacks							
	Time: __ __:__ __						
	Time: __ __:__ __						
	Time: __ __:__ __						
	Time: __ __:__ __						
TOTAL							
Daily Totals							

Water/Fluid Intake ❑❑❑❑❑❑❑❑   *Fruits/Vegetables* ❑❑❑❑❑❑❑❑

Exercise Log

Type	Duration	Calories Burned
TOTAL		

80

Day/Week	Date	Weight

Goals for the Day: _____

Morning	Time: __ __:__ __					Mood	Energy
TOTAL							

Afternoon	Time: __ __:__ __						
TOTAL							

Evening	Time: __ __:__ __						
TOTAL							

Snacks							
	Time: __ __:__ __						
	Time: __ __:__ __						
	Time: __ __:__ __						
	Time: __ __:__ __						
TOTAL							
Daily Totals							

Water/Fluid Intake
❑ ❑ ❑ ❑ ❑ ❑ ❑ ❑

Fruits/Vegetables
❑ ❑ ❑ ❑ ❑ ❑ ❑ ❑

Exercise Log

Type	Duration	Calories Burned
TOTAL		

Day/Week	Date	Weight	*81*

Goals for the Day: _____

Morning	Time: __ __:__ __						Mood	Energy
TOTAL								

Afternoon	Time: __ __:__ __							
TOTAL								

Evening	Time: __ __:__ __							
TOTAL								

Snacks								
Time: __ __:__ __								
Time: __ __:__ __								
Time: __ __:__ __								
Time: __ __:__ __								
TOTAL								
Daily Totals								

Water/Fluid Intake
❑ ❑ ❑ ❑ ❑ ❑ ❑ ❑

Fruits/Vegetables
❑ ❑ ❑ ❑ ❑ ❑ ❑ ❑

Exercise Log

Type	Duration	Calories Burned
TOTAL		

Weekly Assessment

Food Intake Summary

DAY 1				
DAY 2				
DAY 3				
DAY 4				
DAY 5				
DAY 6				
DAY 7				
Weekly Total				
Average Daily Intake (Total ÷ 7)				

Did you meet your goals for water and fruit and veggie intake this week?   Yes   No

Exercise Summary

	Type	Duration	Calories Burned
DAY 1			
DAY 2			
DAY 3			
DAY 4			
DAY 5			
DAY 6			
DAY 7			
TOTALS			

Notes & Gold Star Moments

_____
_____
_____
_____
_____
_____
_____
_____
_____
_____
_____
_____

Goals for Next Week

Eating: _____
_____
_____
_____
_____

Exercise: _____
_____
_____

Other: _____
_____

Day/Week	Date	Weight

Goals for the Day: _____

Morning	Time: __ __:__ __					Mood	Energy
TOTAL							

Afternoon	Time: __ __:__ __						
TOTAL							

Evening	Time: __ __:__ __						
TOTAL							

Snacks							
Time: __ __:__ __							
Time: __ __:__ __							
Time: __ __:__ __							
Time: __ __:__ __							
TOTAL							

Daily Totals							

Water/Fluid Intake
☐ ☐ ☐ ☐ ☐ ☐ ☐ ☐

Fruits/Vegetables
☐ ☐ ☐ ☐ ☐ ☐ ☐ ☐

Exercise Log

Type	Duration	Calories Burned
TOTAL		

84

Goals for the Day: _____

Morning	Time: __ __:__ __					Mood	Energy
TOTAL							

Afternoon	Time: __ __:__ __						
TOTAL							

Evening	Time: __ __:__ __						
TOTAL							

Snacks							
	Time: __ __:__ __						
	Time: __ __:__ __						
	Time: __ __:__ __						
	Time: __ __:__ __						
TOTAL							

Daily Totals							

Water/Fluid Intake
☐ ☐ ☐ ☐ ☐ ☐ ☐ ☐

Fruits/Vegetables
☐ ☐ ☐ ☐ ☐ ☐ ☐ ☐

Exercise Log

Type	Duration	Calories Burned
TOTAL		

Day/Week	Date	Weight	*85*

Goals for the Day: _____

Morning	Time: __ __:__ __					Mood	Energy
TOTAL							
Afternoon	Time: __ __:__ __						
TOTAL							
Evening	Time: __ __:__ __						
TOTAL							
Snacks							
	Time: __ __:__ __						
	Time: __ __:__ __						
	Time: __ __:__ __						
	Time: __ __:__ __						
TOTAL							
Daily Totals							

Water/Fluid Intake
❑ ❑ ❑ ❑ ❑ ❑ ❑ ❑

Fruits/Vegetables
❑ ❑ ❑ ❑ ❑ ❑ ❑ ❑

Exercise Log

Type	Duration	Calories Burned
TOTAL		

86

Day/Week	Date	Weight

Goals for the Day: _____

Morning	Time: __ __:__ __						Mood	Energy
TOTAL								
Afternoon	Time: __ __:__ __							
TOTAL								
Evening	Time: __ __:__ __							
TOTAL								
Snacks								
	Time: __ __:__ __							
	Time: __ __:__ __							
	Time: __ __:__ __							
	Time: __ __:__ __							
TOTAL								
Daily Totals								

Water/Fluid Intake
❏ ❏ ❏ ❏ ❏ ❏ ❏ ❏

Fruits/Vegetables
❏ ❏ ❏ ❏ ❏ ❏ ❏ ❏

Exercise Log

Type	Duration	Calories Burned
TOTAL		

Day/Week	Date	Weight	**87**

Goals for the Day: _____

Morning	Time: __ __:__ __					Mood	Energy
TOTAL							

Afternoon	Time: __ __:__ __						
TOTAL							

Evening	Time: __ __:__ __						
TOTAL							

Snacks							
	Time: __ __:__ __						
	Time: __ __:__ __						
	Time: __ __:__ __						
	Time: __ __:__ __						
TOTAL							

Daily Totals							

Water/Fluid Intake
☐ ☐ ☐ ☐ ☐ ☐ ☐ ☐

Fruits/Vegetables
☐ ☐ ☐ ☐ ☐ ☐ ☐ ☐

Exercise Log

Type	Duration	Calories Burned
TOTAL		

88

Day/Week	Date	Weight

Goals for the Day: _____

Morning	Time: __ __:__ __					Mood	Energy
TOTAL							
Afternoon	Time: __ __:__ __						
TOTAL							
Evening	Time: __ __:__ __						
TOTAL							
Snacks							
	Time: __ __:__ __						
	Time: __ __:__ __						
	Time: __ __:__ __						
	Time: __ __:__ __						
TOTAL							
Daily Totals							

Water/Fluid Intake
❑ ❑ ❑ ❑ ❑ ❑ ❑ ❑

Fruits/Vegetables
❑ ❑ ❑ ❑ ❑ ❑ ❑ ❑

Exercise Log

Type	Duration	Calories Burned
TOTAL		

Day/Week	Date	Weight	

Goals for the Day: _____

Morning	Time: __ __:__ __						Mood	Energy
TOTAL								
Afternoon	Time: __ __:__ __							
TOTAL								
Evening	Time: __ __:__ __							
TOTAL								
Snacks								
	Time: __ __:__ __							
	Time: __ __:__ __							
	Time: __ __:__ __							
	Time: __ __:__ __							
TOTAL								
Daily Totals								

Water/Fluid Intake
☐ ☐ ☐ ☐ ☐ ☐ ☐ ☐

Fruits/Vegetables
☐ ☐ ☐ ☐ ☐ ☐ ☐ ☐

Exercise Log

Type	Duration	Calories Burned
TOTAL		

Weekly Assessment

Food Intake Summary

DAY 1				
DAY 2				
DAY 3				
DAY 4				
DAY 5				
DAY 6				
DAY 7				
Weekly Total				
Average Daily Intake (Total ÷ 7)				

Did you meet your goals for water and fruit and veggie intake this week?   Yes   No

Exercise Summary

	Type	Duration	Calories Burned
DAY 1			
DAY 2			
DAY 3			
DAY 4			
DAY 5			
DAY 6			
DAY 7			
TOTALS			

Notes & Gold Star Moments

_____
_____
_____
_____
_____
_____
_____
_____
_____
_____
_____

Goals for Next Week

Eating:
_____
_____
_____
_____

Exercise:
_____
_____
_____

Other:
_____
_____

Day/Week	Date	Weight	91

Goals for the Day: _____

Morning Time: __ __:__ __						Mood	Energy
TOTAL							
Afternoon Time: __ __:__ __							
TOTAL							
Evening Time: __ __:__ __							
TOTAL							
Snacks							
Time: __ __:__ __							
Time: __ __:__ __							
Time: __ __:__ __							
Time: __ __:__ __							
TOTAL							
Daily Totals							

Water/Fluid Intake
▢ ▢ ▢ ▢ ▢ ▢ ▢ ▢

Fruits/Vegetables
▢ ▢ ▢ ▢ ▢ ▢ ▢ ▢

Exercise Log

Type	Duration	Calories Burned
TOTAL		

92

Goals for the Day: _____

Morning	Time: __ __:__ __						Mood	Energy
TOTAL								

Afternoon	Time: __ __:__ __							
TOTAL								

Evening	Time: __ __:__ __							
TOTAL								

Snacks								
	Time: __ __:__ __							
	Time: __ __:__ __							
	Time: __ __:__ __							
	Time: __ __:__ __							
TOTAL								
Daily Totals								

Water/Fluid Intake
❑ ❑ ❑ ❑ ❑ ❑ ❑ ❑

Fruits/Vegetables
❑ ❑ ❑ ❑ ❑ ❑ ❑ ❑

Exercise Log

Type	Duration	Calories Burned
TOTAL		

Day/Week	Date	Weight	93

Goals for the Day: _____

Morning	Time: __ __:__ __						Mood	Energy
TOTAL								
Afternoon	Time: __ __:__ __							
TOTAL								
Evening	Time: __ __:__ __							
TOTAL								
Snacks								
	Time: __ __:__ __							
	Time: __ __:__ __							
	Time: __ __:__ __							
	Time: __ __:__ __							
TOTAL								
Daily Totals								

Water/Fluid Intake
❑ ❑ ❑ ❑ ❑ ❑ ❑ ❑

Fruits/Vegetables
❑ ❑ ❑ ❑ ❑ ❑ ❑ ❑

Exercise Log

Type	Duration	Calories Burned
TOTAL		

94

Day/Week	Date	Weight

Goals for the Day: _____

Morning	Time: __ __:__ __					Mood	Energy
TOTAL							
Afternoon	Time: __ __:__ __						
TOTAL							
Evening	Time: __ __:__ __						
TOTAL							
Snacks							
	Time: __ __:__ __						
	Time: __ __:__ __						
	Time: __ __:__ __						
	Time: __ __:__ __						
TOTAL							
Daily Totals							

Water/Fluid Intake
❑ ❑ ❑ ❑ ❑ ❑ ❑ ❑ ❑

Fruits/Vegetables
❑ ❑ ❑ ❑ ❑ ❑ ❑ ❑

Exercise Log

Type	Duration	Calories Burned
TOTAL		

Day/Week	Date	Weight

95

Goals for the Day: _____

Morning Time: __ __:__ __						Mood	Energy
TOTAL							
Afternoon Time: __ __:__ __							
TOTAL							
Evening Time: __ __:__ __							
TOTAL							
Snacks							
Time: __ __:__ __							
Time: __ __:__ __							
Time: __ __:__ __							
Time: __ __:__ __							
TOTAL							
Daily Totals							

Water/Fluid Intake
☐ ☐ ☐ ☐ ☐ ☐ ☐ ☐

Fruits/Vegetables
☐ ☐ ☐ ☐ ☐ ☐ ☐ ☐

Exercise Log

Type	Duration	Calories Burned
TOTAL		

96

Day/Week	Date	Weight

Goals for the Day: _____

Morning	Time: __ __:__ __					Mood	Energy
TOTAL							
Afternoon	Time: __ __:__ __						
TOTAL							
Evening	Time: __ __:__ __						
TOTAL							
Snacks							
	Time: __ __:__ __						
	Time: __ __:__ __						
	Time: __ __:__ __						
	Time: __ __:__ __						
TOTAL							
Daily Totals							

Water/Fluid Intake
❑ ❑ ❑ ❑ ❑ ❑ ❑ ❑

Fruits/Vegetables
❑ ❑ ❑ ❑ ❑ ❑ ❑ ❑

Exercise Log

Type	Duration	Calories Burned
TOTAL		

Day/Week	Date	Weight

Goals for the Day: _____

Morning	Time: __ __:__ __						Mood	Energy
TOTAL								
Afternoon	Time: __ __:__ __							
TOTAL								
Evening	Time: __ __:__ __							
TOTAL								
Snacks								
	Time: __ __:__ __							
	Time: __ __:__ __							
	Time: __ __:__ __							
	Time: __ __:__ __							
TOTAL								
Daily Totals								

Water/Fluid Intake
☐ ☐ ☐ ☐ ☐ ☐ ☐ ☐

Fruits/Vegetables
☐ ☐ ☐ ☐ ☐ ☐ ☐ ☐

Exercise Log

Type	Duration	Calories Burned
TOTAL		

Weekly Assessment

Food Intake Summary

DAY 1				
DAY 2				
DAY 3				
DAY 4				
DAY 5				
DAY 6				
DAY 7				
Weekly Total				
Average Daily Intake (Total ÷ 7)				

Did you meet your goals for water and fruit and veggie intake this week?   Yes   No

Exercise Summary

	Type	Duration	Calories Burned
DAY 1			
DAY 2			
DAY 3			
DAY 4			
DAY 5			
DAY 6			
DAY 7			
TOTALS			

Notes & Gold Star Moments

_____
_____
_____
_____
_____
_____
_____
_____
_____
_____
_____
_____

Goals for Next Week

Eating: _____
_____
_____
_____
_____

Exercise: _____
_____
_____

Other: _____
_____

Day/Week	Date	Weight	**99**

Goals for the Day: _____

Morning	Time: __ __:__ __						Mood	Energy
TOTAL								

Afternoon	Time: __ __:__ __							
TOTAL								

Evening	Time: __ __:__ __							
TOTAL								

Snacks								
	Time: __ __:__ __							
	Time: __ __:__ __							
	Time: __ __:__ __							
	Time: __ __:__ __							
TOTAL								

Daily Totals								

Water/Fluid Intake
❑ ❑ ❑ ❑ ❑ ❑ ❑ ❑

Fruits/Vegetables
❑ ❑ ❑ ❑ ❑ ❑ ❑ ❑

Exercise Log

Type	Duration	Calories Burned
TOTAL		

100

Day/Week	Date	Weight

Goals for the Day: _____

Morning	Time: __ __:__ __					Mood	Energy
TOTAL							
Afternoon	Time: __ __:__ __						
TOTAL							
Evening	Time: __ __:__ __						
TOTAL							
Snacks							
	Time: __ __:__ __						
	Time: __ __:__ __						
	Time: __ __:__ __						
	Time: __ __:__ __						
TOTAL							
Daily Totals							

Water/Fluid Intake
❑ ❑ ❑ ❑ ❑ ❑ ❑ ❑

Fruits/Vegetables
❑ ❑ ❑ ❑ ❑ ❑ ❑ ❑

Exercise Log

Type	Duration	Calories Burned
TOTAL		

Day/Week	Date	Weight

Goals for the Day: _____

Morning	Time: __ __:__ __					Mood	Energy
TOTAL							

Afternoon	Time: __ __:__ __						
TOTAL							

Evening	Time: __ __:__ __						
TOTAL							

Snacks							
	Time: __ __:__ __						
	Time: __ __:__ __						
	Time: __ __:__ __						
	Time: __ __:__ __						
TOTAL							
Daily Totals							

Water/Fluid Intake
❏ ❏ ❏ ❏ ❏ ❏ ❏ ❏

Fruits/Vegetables
❏ ❏ ❏ ❏ ❏ ❏ ❏ ❏

Exercise Log

Type	Duration	Calories Burned
TOTAL		

102

Goals for the Day: _____

Morning	Time: __ __:__ __					Mood	Energy
TOTAL							
Afternoon	Time: __ __:__ __						
TOTAL							
Evening	Time: __ __:__ __						
TOTAL							
Snacks							
	Time: __ __:__ __						
	Time: __ __:__ __						
	Time: __ __:__ __						
	Time: __ __:__ __						
TOTAL							
Daily Totals							

Water/Fluid Intake
❏ ❏ ❏ ❏ ❏ ❏ ❏ ❏ ❏

Fruits/Vegetables
❏ ❏ ❏ ❏ ❏ ❏ ❏ ❏

Exercise Log

Type	Duration	Calories Burned
TOTAL		

| Day/Week | Date | Weight | *103* |

Goals for the Day: _____

Morning	Time: __ __:__ __						Mood	Energy
TOTAL								
Afternoon	Time: __ __:__ __							
TOTAL								
Evening	Time: __ __:__ __							
TOTAL								
Snacks								
	Time: __ __:__ __							
	Time: __ __:__ __							
	Time: __ __:__ __							
	Time: __ __:__ __							
TOTAL								
Daily Totals								

Water/Fluid Intake
❑ ❑ ❑ ❑ ❑ ❑ ❑ ❑

Fruits/Vegetables
❑ ❑ ❑ ❑ ❑ ❑ ❑ ❑

Exercise Log

Type	Duration	Calories Burned
TOTAL		

104

Goals for the Day: _____

Morning	Time: __ __:__ __					Mood	Energy
TOTAL							
Afternoon	Time: __ __:__ __						
TOTAL							
Evening	Time: __ __:__ __						
TOTAL							
Snacks							
	Time: __ __:__ __						
	Time: __ __:__ __						
	Time: __ __:__ __						
	Time: __ __:__ __						
TOTAL							
Daily Totals								

Water/Fluid Intake
❑ ❑ ❑ ❑ ❑ ❑ ❑ ❑

Fruits/Vegetables
❑ ❑ ❑ ❑ ❑ ❑ ❑ ❑

Exercise Log

Type	Duration	Calories Burned
TOTAL		

Day/Week	Date	Weight

Goals for the Day: _____

Morning	Time: __ __:__ __					Mood	Energy
TOTAL							

Afternoon	Time: __ __:__ __						
TOTAL							

Evening	Time: __ __:__ __						
TOTAL							

Snacks							
	Time: __ __:__ __						
	Time: __ __:__ __						
	Time: __ __:__ __						
	Time: __ __:__ __						
TOTAL							
Daily Totals							

Water/Fluid Intake
☐ ☐ ☐ ☐ ☐ ☐ ☐ ☐

Fruits/Vegetables
☐ ☐ ☐ ☐ ☐ ☐ ☐ ☐

Exercise Log

Type	Duration	Calories Burned
TOTAL		

Weekly Assessment

Food Intake Summary

DAY 1				
DAY 2				
DAY 3				
DAY 4				
DAY 5				
DAY 6				
DAY 7				
Weekly Total				
Average Daily Intake (Total ÷ 7)				

Did you meet your goals for water and fruit and veggie intake this week?   Yes   No

Exercise Summary

	Type	Duration	Calories Burned
DAY 1			
DAY 2			
DAY 3			
DAY 4			
DAY 5			
DAY 6			
DAY 7			
TOTALS			

Notes & Gold Star Moments

_____

_____

_____

_____

_____

_____

_____

_____

_____

_____

_____

Goals for Next Week

Eating: _____

_____

_____

_____

Exercise: _____

_____

_____

Other: _____

_____

Day/Week	Date	Weight	**107**

Goals for the Day: _____

Morning	Time: __ __:__ __						Mood	Energy
TOTAL								

Afternoon	Time: __ __:__ __							
TOTAL								

Evening	Time: __ __:__ __							
TOTAL								

Snacks								
	Time: __ __:__ __							
	Time: __ __:__ __							
	Time: __ __:__ __							
	Time: __ __:__ __							
TOTAL								
Daily Totals								

Water/Fluid Intake
❏ ❏ ❏ ❏ ❏ ❏ ❏ ❏

Fruits/Vegetables
❏ ❏ ❏ ❏ ❏ ❏ ❏ ❏

Exercise Log

Type	Duration	Calories Burned
TOTAL		

108

Day/Week	Date	Weight

Goals for the Day: _____

Morning	Time: __ __:__ __						Mood	Energy
TOTAL								

Afternoon	Time: __ __:__ __							
TOTAL								

Evening	Time: __ __:__ __							
TOTAL								

Snacks								
	Time: __ __:__ __							
	Time: __ __:__ __							
	Time: __ __:__ __							
	Time: __ __:__ __							
TOTAL								
Daily Totals								

Water/Fluid Intake
❑ ❑ ❑ ❑ ❑ ❑ ❑

Fruits/Vegetables
❑ ❑ ❑ ❑ ❑ ❑ ❑ ❑

Exercise Log

Type	Duration	Calories Burned
TOTAL		

Day/Week	Date	Weight	109

Goals for the Day: _____

Morning	Time: __ __:__ __						Mood	Energy
TOTAL								

Afternoon	Time: __ __:__ __							
TOTAL								

Evening	Time: __ __:__ __							
TOTAL								

Snacks								
	Time: __ __:__ __							
	Time: __ __:__ __							
	Time: __ __:__ __							
	Time: __ __:__ __							
TOTAL								
Daily Totals								

Water/Fluid Intake
❑ ❑ ❑ ❑ ❑ ❑ ❑ ❑

Fruits/Vegetables
❑ ❑ ❑ ❑ ❑ ❑ ❑ ❑

Exercise Log

Type	Duration	Calories Burned
TOTAL		

Day/Week	Date	Weight

Goals for the Day: _____

Morning	Time: __ __ : __ __					Mood	Energy
TOTAL							

Afternoon	Time: __ __ : __ __						
TOTAL							

Evening	Time: __ __ : __ __						
TOTAL							

Snacks							
	Time: __ __ : __ __						
	Time: __ __ : __ __						
	Time: __ __ : __ __						
	Time: __ __ : __ __						
TOTAL							
Daily Totals							

Water/Fluid Intake
❑ ❑ ❑ ❑ ❑ ❑ ❑ ❑

Fruits/Vegetables
❑ ❑ ❑ ❑ ❑ ❑ ❑ ❑

Exercise Log

Type	Duration	Calories Burned
TOTAL		

Day/Week	Date	Weight

Goals for the Day: _____

Morning	Time: __ __:__ __					Mood	Energy
TOTAL							
Afternoon	Time: __ __:__ __						
TOTAL							
Evening	Time: __ __:__ __						
TOTAL							
Snacks							
	Time: __ __:__ __						
	Time: __ __:__ __						
	Time: __ __:__ __						
	Time: __ __:__ __						
TOTAL							
Daily Totals							

Water/Fluid Intake
❑ ❑ ❑ ❑ ❑ ❑ ❑ ❑

Fruits/Vegetables
❑ ❑ ❑ ❑ ❑ ❑ ❑ ❑

Exercise Log

Type	Duration	Calories Burned
TOTAL		

112

Day/Week	Date	Weight

Goals for the Day: _____

Morning	Time: __ __:__ __					Mood	Energy
TOTAL							
Afternoon	Time: __ __:__ __						
TOTAL							
Evening	Time: __ __:__ __						
TOTAL							
Snacks							
	Time: __ __:__ __						
	Time: __ __:__ __						
	Time: __ __:__ __						
	Time: __ __:__ __						
TOTAL							
Daily Totals							

Water/Fluid Intake
☐ ☐ ☐ ☐ ☐ ☐ ☐ ☐

Fruits/Vegetables
☐ ☐ ☐ ☐ ☐ ☐ ☐ ☐

Exercise Log

Type	Duration	Calories Burned
TOTAL		

Day/Week	Date	Weight	*113*

Goals for the Day: _____

Morning	Time: __ __:__ __						Mood	Energy
TOTAL								

Afternoon	Time: __ __:__ __							
TOTAL								

Evening	Time: __ __:__ __							
TOTAL								

Snacks								
	Time: __ __:__ __							
	Time: __ __:__ __							
	Time: __ __:__ __							
	Time: __ __:__ __							
TOTAL								
Daily Totals								

Water/Fluid Intake
❑ ❑ ❑ ❑ ❑ ❑ ❑ ❑

Fruits/Vegetables
❑ ❑ ❑ ❑ ❑ ❑ ❑ ❑

Exercise Log

Type	Duration	Calories Burned
TOTAL		

Food Intake Summary

DAY 1				
DAY 2				
DAY 3				
DAY 4				
DAY 5				
DAY 6				
DAY 7				
Weekly Total				
Average Daily Intake (Total ÷ 7)				

Did you meet your goals for water and fruit and veggie intake this week?   Yes   No

Exercise Summary

	Type	Duration	Calories Burned
DAY 1			
DAY 2			
DAY 3			
DAY 4			
DAY 5			
DAY 6			
DAY 7			
TOTALS			

Notes & Gold Star Moments

_____
_____
_____
_____
_____
_____
_____
_____
_____
_____
_____
_____

Goals for Next Week

Eating: _____
_____
_____
_____
_____

Exercise: _____
_____
_____

Other: _____
_____

Goals for the Day: _____

Morning	Time: __ __ : __ __						Mood	Energy
TOTAL								
Afternoon	Time: __ __ : __ __							
TOTAL								
Evening	Time: __ __ : __ __							
TOTAL								
Snacks								
	Time: __ __ : __ __							
	Time: __ __ : __ __							
	Time: __ __ : __ __							
	Time: __ __ : __ __							
TOTAL								
Daily Totals								

Water/Fluid Intake
❏ ❏ ❏ ❏ ❏ ❏ ❏

Fruits/Vegetables
❏ ❏ ❏ ❏ ❏ ❏ ❏

Exercise Log

Type	Duration	Calories Burned
TOTAL		

116

Goals for the Day: _____

Morning	Time: __ __:__ __						Mood	Energy
TOTAL								
Afternoon	Time: __ __:__ __							
TOTAL								
Evening	Time: __ __:__ __							
TOTAL								
Snacks								
	Time: __ __:__ __							
	Time: __ __:__ __							
	Time: __ __:__ __							
	Time: __ __:__ __							
TOTAL								
Daily Totals								

Water/Fluid Intake
❑ ❑ ❑ ❑ ❑ ❑ ❑ ❑

Fruits/Vegetables
❑ ❑ ❑ ❑ ❑ ❑ ❑ ❑

Exercise Log

Type	Duration	Calories Burned
TOTAL		

Day/Week	Date	Weight	117

Goals for the Day: _____

Morning	Time: __ __:__ __					Mood	Energy
TOTAL							

Afternoon	Time: __ __:__ __						
TOTAL							

Evening	Time: __ __:__ __						
TOTAL							

Snacks							
	Time: __ __:__ __						
	Time: __ __:__ __						
	Time: __ __:__ __						
	Time: __ __:__ __						
TOTAL							
Daily Totals							

Water/Fluid Intake
☐ ☐ ☐ ☐ ☐ ☐ ☐ ☐

Fruits/Vegetables
☐ ☐ ☐ ☐ ☐ ☐ ☐ ☐

Exercise Log

Type	Duration	Calories Burned
TOTAL		

118

Goals for the Day: _____

Morning	Time: __ __:__ __					Mood	Energy
TOTAL							
Afternoon	Time: __ __:__ __						
TOTAL							
Evening	Time: __ __:__ __						
TOTAL							
Snacks							
	Time: __ __:__ __						
	Time: __ __:__ __						
	Time: __ __:__ __						
	Time: __ __:__ __						
TOTAL							
Daily Totals							

Water/Fluid Intake
☐ ☐ ☐ ☐ ☐ ☐ ☐

Fruits/Vegetables
☐ ☐ ☐ ☐ ☐ ☐ ☐ ☐

Exercise Log

Type	Duration	Calories Burned
TOTAL		

| Day/Week | Date | Weight | **119** |

Goals for the Day: _____

Morning	Time: __ __:__ __					Mood	Energy
TOTAL							
Afternoon	Time: __ __:__ __						
TOTAL							
Evening	Time: __ __:__ __						
TOTAL							
Snacks							
	Time: __ __:__ __						
	Time: __ __:__ __						
	Time: __ __:__ __						
	Time: __ __:__ __						
TOTAL							
Daily Totals							

Water/Fluid Intake
❑ ❑ ❑ ❑ ❑ ❑ ❑ ❑

Fruits/Vegetables
❑ ❑ ❑ ❑ ❑ ❑ ❑ ❑

Exercise Log

Type	Duration	Calories Burned
TOTAL		

120

Day/Week	Date	Weight

Goals for the Day: _____

Morning	Time: __ __ : __ __					Mood	Energy
TOTAL							
Afternoon	Time: __ __ : __ __						
TOTAL							
Evening	Time: __ __ : __ __						
TOTAL							
Snacks							
	Time: __ __ : __ __						
	Time: __ __ : __ __						
	Time: __ __ : __ __						
	Time: __ __ : __ __						
TOTAL							
Daily Totals							

Water/Fluid Intake
☐ ☐ ☐ ☐ ☐ ☐ ☐ ☐

Fruits/Vegetables
☐ ☐ ☐ ☐ ☐ ☐ ☐ ☐

Exercise Log

Type	Duration	Calories Burned
TOTAL		

Day/Week	Date	Weight

Goals for the Day: _____

Morning	Time: __ __:__ __						Mood	Energy
TOTAL								
Afternoon	Time: __ __:__ __							
TOTAL								
Evening	Time: __ __:__ __							
TOTAL								
Snacks								
	Time: __ __:__ __							
	Time: __ __:__ __							
	Time: __ __:__ __							
	Time: __ __:__ __							
TOTAL								
Daily Totals								

Water/Fluid Intake
❑ ❑ ❑ ❑ ❑ ❑ ❑ ❑

Fruits/Vegetables
❑ ❑ ❑ ❑ ❑ ❑ ❑ ❑

Exercise Log

Type	Duration	Calories Burned
TOTAL		

122 *Weekly Assessment*

Food Intake Summary

DAY 1				
DAY 2				
DAY 3				
DAY 4				
DAY 5				
DAY 6				
DAY 7				
Weekly Total				
Average Daily Intake (Total ÷ 7)				

Did you meet your goals for water and fruit and veggie intake this week?   Yes   No

Exercise Summary

	Type	Duration	Calories Burned
DAY 1			
DAY 2			
DAY 3			
DAY 4			
DAY 5			
DAY 6			
DAY 7			
TOTALS			

Notes & Gold Star Moments

Goals for Next Week

Eating:

Exercise:

Other:

Day/Week	Date	Weight	**123**

Goals for the Day: _____

Morning	Time: __ __:__ __					Mood	Energy
TOTAL							

Afternoon	Time: __ __:__ __						
TOTAL							

Evening	Time: __ __:__ __						
TOTAL							

Snacks							
	Time: __ __:__ __						
	Time: __ __:__ __						
	Time: __ __:__ __						
	Time: __ __:__ __						
TOTAL							
Daily Totals							

Water/Fluid Intake
❏ ❏ ❏ ❏ ❏ ❏ ❏ ❏

Fruits/Vegetables
❏ ❏ ❏ ❏ ❏ ❏ ❏ ❏

Exercise Log

Type	Duration	Calories Burned
TOTAL		

124

Day/Week	Date	Weight

Goals for the Day: _____

Morning Time: __ __:__ __						Mood	Energy
TOTAL							
Afternoon Time: __ __:__ __							
TOTAL							
Evening Time: __ __:__ __							
TOTAL							
Snacks							
Time: __ __:__ __							
Time: __ __:__ __							
Time: __ __:__ __							
Time: __ __:__ __							
TOTAL							
Daily Totals							

Water/Fluid Intake
❏ ❏ ❏ ❏ ❏ ❏ ❏

Fruits/Vegetables
❏ ❏ ❏ ❏ ❏ ❏ ❏

Exercise Log

Type	Duration	Calories Burned
TOTAL		

Day/Week	Date	Weight

Goals for the Day: _____

Morning	Time: __ __:__ __					Mood	Energy
TOTAL							
Afternoon	Time: __ __:__ __						
TOTAL							
Evening	Time: __ __:__ __						
TOTAL							
Snacks							
	Time: __ __:__ __						
	Time: __ __:__ __						
	Time: __ __:__ __						
	Time: __ __:__ __						
TOTAL							
Daily Totals							

Water/Fluid Intake
❑ ❑ ❑ ❑ ❑ ❑ ❑ ❑

Fruits/Vegetables
❑ ❑ ❑ ❑ ❑ ❑ ❑ ❑

Exercise Log

Type	Duration	Calories Burned
TOTAL		

126

Day/Week	Date	Weight

Goals for the Day: _____

Morning	Time: __ __:__ __					Mood	Energy
TOTAL							
Afternoon	Time: __ __:__ __						
TOTAL							
Evening	Time: __ __:__ __						
TOTAL							
Snacks							
	Time: __ __:__ __						
	Time: __ __:__ __						
	Time: __ __:__ __						
	Time: __ __:__ __						
TOTAL							
Daily Totals							

Water/Fluid Intake
❑ ❑ ❑ ❑ ❑ ❑ ❑ ❑

Fruits/Vegetables
❑ ❑ ❑ ❑ ❑ ❑ ❑ ❑

Exercise Log

Type	Duration	Calories Burned
TOTAL		

Day/Week	Date	Weight	**127**

Goals for the Day: _____

Morning	Time: __ __:__ __					Mood	Energy
TOTAL							
Afternoon	Time: __ __:__ __						
TOTAL							
Evening	Time: __ __:__ __						
TOTAL							
Snacks							
	Time: __ __:__ __						
	Time: __ __:__ __						
	Time: __ __:__ __						
	Time: __ __:__ __						
TOTAL							
Daily Totals							

Water/Fluid Intake
☐☐☐☐☐☐☐☐

Fruits/Vegetables
☐☐☐☐☐☐☐☐

Exercise Log

Type	Duration	Calories Burned
TOTAL		

128

Day/Week	Date	Weight

Goals for the Day: _____

Morning	Time: __ __:__ __						Mood	Energy
TOTAL								
Afternoon	Time: __ __:__ __							
TOTAL								
Evening	Time: __ __:__ __							
TOTAL								
Snacks								
Time: __ __:__ __								
Time: __ __:__ __								
Time: __ __:__ __								
Time: __ __:__ __								
TOTAL								
Daily Totals								

Water/Fluid Intake
❑ ❑ ❑ ❑ ❑ ❑ ❑

Fruits/Vegetables
❑ ❑ ❑ ❑ ❑ ❑ ❑

Exercise Log

Type	Duration	Calories Burned
TOTAL		

Day/Week	Date	Weight

Goals for the Day: _____

Morning	Time: __ __:__ __					Mood	Energy
TOTAL							

Afternoon	Time: __ __:__ __						
TOTAL							

Evening	Time: __ __:__ __						
TOTAL							

Snacks							
	Time: __ __:__ __						
	Time: __ __:__ __						
	Time: __ __:__ __						
	Time: __ __:__ __						
TOTAL							
Daily Totals							

Water/Fluid Intake
❑ ❑ ❑ ❑ ❑ ❑ ❑ ❑

Fruits/Vegetables
❑ ❑ ❑ ❑ ❑ ❑ ❑

Exercise Log

Type	Duration	Calories Burned
TOTAL		

Food Intake Summary

DAY 1				
DAY 2				
DAY 3				
DAY 4				
DAY 5				
DAY 6				
DAY 7				
Weekly Total				
Average Daily Intake (Total ÷ 7)				

Did you meet your goals for water and fruit and veggie intake this week?   Yes   No

Exercise Summary

	Type	Duration	Calories Burned
DAY 1			
DAY 2			
DAY 3			
DAY 4			
DAY 5			
DAY 6			
DAY 7			
TOTALS			

Notes & Gold Star Moments

_____
_____
_____
_____
_____
_____
_____
_____
_____
_____

Goals for Next Week

Eating: _____
_____
_____
_____
_____

Exercise: _____
_____
_____

Other: _____
_____

Day/Week	Date	Weight

Goals for the Day: _____

Morning	Time: __ __:__ __						Mood	Energy
TOTAL								

Afternoon	Time: __ __:__ __							
TOTAL								

Evening	Time: __ __:__ __							
TOTAL								

Snacks								
	Time: __ __:__ __							
	Time: __ __:__ __							
	Time: __ __:__ __							
	Time: __ __:__ __							
TOTAL								
Daily Totals								

Water/Fluid Intake
☐ ☐ ☐ ☐ ☐ ☐ ☐ ☐

Fruits/Vegetables
☐ ☐ ☐ ☐ ☐ ☐ ☐ ☐

Exercise Log

Type	Duration	Calories Burned
TOTAL		

132

Day/Week	Date	Weight

Goals for the Day: _____

Morning	Time: __ __:__ __					Mood	Energy
TOTAL							
Afternoon	Time: __ __:__ __						
TOTAL							
Evening	Time: __ __:__ __						
TOTAL							
Snacks							
	Time: __ __:__ __						
	Time: __ __:__ __						
	Time: __ __:__ __						
	Time: __ __:__ __						
TOTAL							
Daily Totals							

Water/Fluid Intake
❑ ❑ ❑ ❑ ❑ ❑ ❑ ❑

Fruits/Vegetables
❑ ❑ ❑ ❑ ❑ ❑ ❑ ❑

Exercise Log

Type	Duration	Calories Burned
TOTAL		

Day/Week	Date	Weight

Goals for the Day: _____

Morning	Time: __ __:__ __						Mood	Energy
TOTAL								

Afternoon	Time: __ __:__ __							
TOTAL								

Evening	Time: __ __:__ __							
TOTAL								

Snacks								
	Time: __ __:__ __							
	Time: __ __:__ __							
	Time: __ __:__ __							
	Time: __ __:__ __							
TOTAL								
Daily Totals								

Water/Fluid Intake
❑ ❑ ❑ ❑ ❑ ❑ ❑ ❑

Fruits/Vegetables
❑ ❑ ❑ ❑ ❑ ❑ ❑ ❑

Exercise Log

Type	Duration	Calories Burned
TOTAL		

134

Day/Week	Date	Weight

Goals for the Day: _____

Morning	Time: __ __:__ __					Mood	Energy
TOTAL							
Afternoon	Time: __ __:__ __						
TOTAL							
Evening	Time: __ __:__ __						
TOTAL							
Snacks							
	Time: __ __:__ __						
	Time: __ __:__ __						
	Time: __ __:__ __						
	Time: __ __:__ __						
TOTAL							
Daily Totals							

Water/Fluid Intake
❏ ❏ ❏ ❏ ❏ ❏ ❏ ❏

Fruits/Vegetables
❏ ❏ ❏ ❏ ❏ ❏ ❏ ❏

Exercise Log

Type	Duration	Calories Burned
TOTAL		

Day/Week	Date	Weight	**135**

Goals for the Day: _____

Morning	Time: __ __:__ __						Mood	Energy
	TOTAL							
Afternoon	Time: __ __:__ __							
	TOTAL							
Evening	Time: __ __:__ __							
	TOTAL							
Snacks								
	Time: __ __:__ __							
	Time: __ __:__ __							
	Time: __ __:__ __							
	Time: __ __:__ __							
	TOTAL							
Daily Totals								

Water/Fluid Intake
❑ ❑ ❑ ❑ ❑ ❑ ❑ ❑

Fruits/Vegetables
❑ ❑ ❑ ❑ ❑ ❑ ❑ ❑

Exercise Log

Type	Duration	Calories Burned
TOTAL		

Day/Week	Date	Weight

Goals for the Day: _____

Morning	Time: __ __:__ __					Mood	Energy
TOTAL							
Afternoon	Time: __ __:__ __						
TOTAL							
Evening	Time: __ __:__ __						
TOTAL							
Snacks							
	Time: __ __:__ __						
	Time: __ __:__ __						
	Time: __ __:__ __						
	Time: __ __:__ __						
TOTAL							
Daily Totals							

Water/Fluid Intake
☐ ☐ ☐ ☐ ☐ ☐ ☐ ☐

Fruits/Vegetables
☐ ☐ ☐ ☐ ☐ ☐ ☐ ☐

Exercise Log

Type	Duration	Calories Burned
TOTAL		

Day/Week	Date	Weight	137

Goals for the Day: _____

Morning	Time: __ __:__ __					Mood	Energy
TOTAL							
Afternoon	Time: __ __:__ __						
TOTAL							
Evening	Time: __ __:__ __						
TOTAL							
Snacks							
	Time: __ __:__ __						
	Time: __ __:__ __						
	Time: __ __:__ __						
	Time: __ __:__ __						
TOTAL							
Daily Totals							

Water/Fluid Intake
❑ ❑ ❑ ❑ ❑ ❑ ❑ ❑

Fruits/Vegetables
❑ ❑ ❑ ❑ ❑ ❑ ❑ ❑

Exercise Log

Type	Duration	Calories Burned
TOTAL		

Weekly Assessment

Food Intake Summary

DAY 1				
DAY 2				
DAY 3				
DAY 4				
DAY 5				
DAY 6				
DAY 7				
Weekly Total				
Average Daily Intake (Total ÷ 7)				

Did you meet your goals for water and fruit and veggie intake this week?   Yes   No

Exercise Summary

	Type	Duration	Calories Burned
DAY 1			
DAY 2			
DAY 3			
DAY 4			
DAY 5			
DAY 6			
DAY 7			
TOTALS			

Notes & Gold Star Moments

_____
_____
_____
_____
_____
_____
_____
_____
_____
_____
_____
_____

Goals for Next Week

Eating: _____
_____
_____
_____
_____
_____

Exercise: _____
_____
_____

Other: _____
_____

Day/Week	Date	Weight

Goals for the Day: _____

Morning	Time: __ __ : __ __					Mood	Energy
TOTAL							
Afternoon	Time: __ __ : __ __						
	·						
TOTAL							
Evening	Time: __ __ : __ __						
TOTAL							
Snacks							
	Time: __ __ : __ __						
	Time: __ __ : __ __						
	Time: __ __ : __ __						
	Time: __ __ : __ __						
TOTAL							
Daily Totals							

Water/Fluid Intake
☐ ☐ ☐ ☐ ☐ ☐ ☐ ☐

Fruits/Vegetables
☐ ☐ ☐ ☐ ☐ ☐ ☐ ☐

Exercise Log

Type	Duration	Calories Burned
TOTAL		

140

Day/Week	Date	Weight

Goals for the Day: _____

Morning	Time: __ __:__ __						Mood	Energy
TOTAL								
Afternoon	Time: __ __:__ __							
TOTAL								
Evening	Time: __ __:__ __							
TOTAL								
Snacks								
	Time: __ __:__ __							
	Time: __ __:__ __							
	Time: __ __:__ __							
	Time: __ __:__ __							
TOTAL								
Daily Totals								

Water/Fluid Intake
❑ ❑ ❑ ❑ ❑ ❑ ❑ ❑

Fruits/Vegetables
❑ ❑ ❑ ❑ ❑ ❑ ❑ ❑

Exercise Log

Type	Duration	Calories Burned
TOTAL		

Day/Week	Date	Weight

Goals for the Day: _____

Morning	Time: __ __:__ __					Mood	Energy
TOTAL							
Afternoon	Time: __ __:__ __						
TOTAL							
Evening	Time: __ __:__ __						
TOTAL							
Snacks							
	Time: __ __:__ __						
	Time: __ __:__ __						
	Time: __ __:__ __						
	Time: __ __:__ __						
TOTAL							
Daily Totals							

Water/Fluid Intake
❑ ❑ ❑ ❑ ❑ ❑ ❑ ❑

Fruits/Vegetables
❑ ❑ ❑ ❑ ❑ ❑ ❑ ❑

Exercise Log

Type	Duration	Calories Burned
TOTAL		

142

Day/Week	Date	Weight

Goals for the Day: _____

Morning	Time: __ __:__ __					Mood	Energy
TOTAL							
Afternoon	Time: __ __:__ __						
TOTAL							
Evening	Time: __ __:__ __						
TOTAL							
Snacks							
	Time: __ __:__ __						
	Time: __ __:__ __						
	Time: __ __:__ __						
	Time: __ __:__ __						
TOTAL							
Daily Totals							

Water/Fluid Intake
❑ ❑ ❑ ❑ ❑ ❑ ❑ ❑

Fruits/Vegetables
❑ ❑ ❑ ❑ ❑ ❑ ❑ ❑

Exercise Log

Type	Duration	Calories Burned
TOTAL		

143

Day/Week	Date	Weight

Goals for the Day: _____

Morning	Time: __ __:__ __					Mood	Energy
TOTAL							

Afternoon	Time: __ __:__ __						
TOTAL							

Evening	Time: __ __:__ __						
TOTAL							

Snacks							
	Time: __ __:__ __						
	Time: __ __:__ __						
	Time: __ __:__ __						
	Time: __ __:__ __						
TOTAL							
Daily Totals							

Water/Fluid Intake
☐ ☐ ☐ ☐ ☐ ☐ ☐ ☐

Fruits/Vegetables
☐ ☐ ☐ ☐ ☐ ☐ ☐ ☐

Exercise Log

Type	Duration	Calories Burned
TOTAL		

144

Day/Week	Date	Weight

Goals for the Day: _____

Morning	Time: __ __:__ __					Mood	Energy
TOTAL							
Afternoon	Time: __ __:__ __						
TOTAL							
Evening	Time: __ __:__ __						
TOTAL							
Snacks							
	Time: __ __:__ __						
	Time: __ __:__ __						
	Time: __ __:__ __						
	Time: __ __:__ __						
TOTAL							
Daily Totals							

Water/Fluid Intake
❏ ❏ ❏ ❏ ❏ ❏ ❏ ❏

Fruits/Vegetables
❏ ❏ ❏ ❏ ❏ ❏ ❏ ❏

Exercise Log

Type	Duration	Calories Burned
TOTAL		

Day/Week	Date	Weight

Goals for the Day: _____

Morning	Time: __ __:__ __					Mood	Energy
TOTAL							
Afternoon	Time: __ __:__ __						
TOTAL							
Evening	Time: __ __:__ __						
TOTAL							
Snacks							
	Time: __ __:__ __						
	Time: __ __:__ __						
	Time: __ __:__ __						
	Time: __ __:__ __						
TOTAL							
Daily Totals							

Water/Fluid Intake
❑ ❑ ❑ ❑ ❑ ❑ ❑ ❑

Fruits/Vegetables
❑ ❑ ❑ ❑ ❑ ❑ ❑ ❑

Exercise Log

Type	Duration	Calories Burned
TOTAL		

Food Intake Summary

DAY 1			
DAY 2			
DAY 3			
DAY 4			
DAY 5			
DAY 6			
DAY 7			
Weekly Total			
Average Daily Intake (Total ÷ 7)			

Did you meet your goals for water and fruit and veggie intake this week?   Yes   No

Exercise Summary

	Type	Duration	Calories Burned
DAY 1			
DAY 2			
DAY 3			
DAY 4			
DAY 5			
DAY 6			
DAY 7			
TOTALS			

Notes & Gold Star Moments

Goals for Next Week

Eating:

Exercise:

Other:

Day/Week	Date	Weight	**147**

Goals for the Day: _____

Morning	Time: __ __ : __ __					Mood	Energy
TOTAL							

Afternoon	Time: __ __ : __ __						
TOTAL							

Evening	Time: __ __ : __ __						
TOTAL							

Snacks							
	Time: __ __ : __ __						
	Time: __ __ : __ __						
	Time: __ __ : __ __						
	Time: __ __ : __ __						
TOTAL							
Daily Totals							

Water/Fluid Intake
☐ ☐ ☐ ☐ ☐ ☐ ☐ ☐

Fruits/Vegetables
☐ ☐ ☐ ☐ ☐ ☐ ☐ ☐

Exercise Log

Type	Duration	Calories Burned
TOTAL		

148

Goals for the Day: _____

Morning	Time: __ __:__ __					Mood	Energy
TOTAL							
Afternoon	Time: __ __:__ __						
TOTAL							
Evening	Time: __ __:__ __						
TOTAL							
Snacks							
	Time: __ __:__ __						
	Time: __ __:__ __						
	Time: __ __:__ __						
	Time: __ __:__ __						
TOTAL							
Daily Totals							

Water/Fluid Intake
☐ ☐ ☐ ☐ ☐ ☐ ☐ ☐

Fruits/Vegetables
☐ ☐ ☐ ☐ ☐ ☐ ☐ ☐

Exercise Log

Type	Duration	Calories Burned
TOTAL		

Day/Week	Date	Weight

Goals for the Day: _____

Morning	Time: __ __:__ __						Mood	Energy
TOTAL								

Afternoon	Time: __ __:__ __							
TOTAL								

Evening	Time: __ __:__ __							
TOTAL								

Snacks								
	Time: __ __:__ __							
	Time: __ __:__ __							
	Time: __ __:__ __							
	Time: __ __:__ __							
TOTAL								

Daily Totals								

Water/Fluid Intake
☐ ☐ ☐ ☐ ☐ ☐ ☐ ☐

Fruits/Vegetables
☐ ☐ ☐ ☐ ☐ ☐ ☐ ☐

Exercise Log

Type	Duration	Calories Burned
TOTAL		

150

Goals for the Day: _____

Morning	Time: __ __:__ __					Mood	Energy
	TOTAL						

Afternoon	Time: __ __:__ __						
	TOTAL						

Evening	Time: __ __:__ __						
	TOTAL						

Snacks							
	Time: __ __:__ __						
	Time: __ __:__ __						
	Time: __ __:__ __						
	Time: __ __:__ __						
	TOTAL						
Daily Totals							

Water/Fluid Intake
❑ ❑ ❑ ❑ ❑ ❑ ❑ ❑

Fruits/Vegetables
❑ ❑ ❑ ❑ ❑ ❑ ❑ ❑

Exercise Log

Type	Duration	Calories Burned
TOTAL		

Day/Week	Date	Weight

Goals for the Day: _____

Morning	Time: __ __:__ __					Mood	Energy
TOTAL							
Afternoon	Time: __ __:__ __						
TOTAL							
Evening	Time: __ __:__ __						
TOTAL							
Snacks							
	Time: __ __:__ __						
	Time: __ __:__ __						
	Time: __ __:__ __						
	Time: __ __:__ __						
TOTAL							
Daily Totals							

Water/Fluid Intake
❑ ❑ ❑ ❑ ❑ ❑ ❑ ❑

Fruits/Vegetables
❑ ❑ ❑ ❑ ❑ ❑ ❑ ❑

Exercise Log

Type	Duration	Calories Burned
TOTAL		

152

Goals for the Day: _____

Morning	Time: __ __:__ __						Mood	Energy
TOTAL								
Afternoon	Time: __ __:__ __							
TOTAL								
Evening	Time: __ __:__ __							
TOTAL								
Snacks								
	Time: __ __:__ __							
	Time: __ __:__ __							
	Time: __ __:__ __							
	Time: __ __:__ __							
TOTAL								
Daily Totals								

Water/Fluid Intake
❏ ❏ ❏ ❏ ❏ ❏ ❏ ❏

Fruits/Vegetables
❏ ❏ ❏ ❏ ❏ ❏ ❏ ❏

Exercise Log

Type	Duration	Calories Burned
TOTAL		

Day/Week	Date	Weight

Goals for the Day: _____

Morning	Time: __ __:__ __					Mood	Energy
TOTAL							
Afternoon	Time: __ __:__ __						
TOTAL							
Evening	Time: __ __:__ __						
TOTAL							
Snacks							
	Time: __ __:__ __						
	Time: __ __:__ __						
	Time: __ __:__ __						
	Time: __ __:__ __						
TOTAL							
Daily Totals							

Water/Fluid Intake
❑ ❑ ❑ ❑ ❑ ❑ ❑ ❑

Fruits/Vegetables
❑ ❑ ❑ ❑ ❑ ❑ ❑ ❑

Exercise Log

Type	Duration	Calories Burned
TOTAL		

Weekly Assessment

Food Intake Summary

DAY 1				
DAY 2				
DAY 3				
DAY 4				
DAY 5				
DAY 6				
DAY 7				
Weekly Total				
Average Daily Intake (Total ÷ 7)				

Did you meet your goals for water and fruit and veggie intake this week?   Yes   No

Exercise Summary

	Type	Duration	Calories Burned
DAY 1			
DAY 2			
DAY 3			
DAY 4			
DAY 5			
DAY 6			
DAY 7			
TOTALS			

Notes & Gold Star Moments

Goals for Next Week

Eating:

Exercise:

Other:

Day/Week	Date	Weight

Goals for the Day: _____

Morning	Time: __ __:__ __						Mood	Energy
TOTAL								
Afternoon	Time: __ __:__ __							
TOTAL								
Evening	Time: __ __:__ __							
TOTAL								
Snacks								
	Time: __ __:__ __							
	Time: __ __:__ __							
	Time: __ __:__ __							
	Time: __ __:__ __							
TOTAL								
Daily Totals								

Water/Fluid Intake
☐ ☐ ☐ ☐ ☐ ☐ ☐ ☐

Fruits/Vegetables
☐ ☐ ☐ ☐ ☐ ☐ ☐ ☐

Exercise Log

Type	Duration	Calories Burned
TOTAL		

156

Day/Week	Date	Weight

Goals for the Day: _____

Morning	Time: __ __:__ __					Mood	Energy
TOTAL							
Afternoon	Time: __ __:__ __						
TOTAL							
Evening	Time: __ __:__ __						
TOTAL							
Snacks							
	Time: __ __:__ __						
	Time: __ __:__ __						
	Time: __ __:__ __						
	Time: __ __:__ __						
TOTAL							
Daily Totals							

Water/Fluid Intake
❑ ❑ ❑ ❑ ❑ ❑ ❑ ❑

Fruits/Vegetables
❑ ❑ ❑ ❑ ❑ ❑ ❑ ❑

Exercise Log

Type	Duration	Calories Burned
TOTAL		

Day/Week	Date	Weight	

Goals for the Day: _____

Morning	Time: __ __:__ __					Mood	Energy
TOTAL							
Afternoon	Time: __ __:__ __						
TOTAL							
Evening	Time: __ __:__ __						
TOTAL							
Snacks							
	Time: __ __:__ __						
	Time: __ __:__ __						
	Time: __ __:__ __						
	Time: __ __:__ __						
TOTAL							
Daily Totals							

Water/Fluid Intake
❑ ❑ ❑ ❑ ❑ ❑ ❑ ❑

Fruits/Vegetables
❑ ❑ ❑ ❑ ❑ ❑ ❑ ❑

Exercise Log

Type	Duration	Calories Burned
TOTAL		

158

Day/Week	Date	Weight

Goals for the Day: _____

Morning Time: __ __:__ __					Mood	Energy
TOTAL						
Afternoon Time: __ __:__ __						
TOTAL						
Evening Time: __ __:__ __						
TOTAL						
Snacks						
Time: __ __:__ __						
Time: __ __:__ __						
Time: __ __:__ __						
Time: __ __:__ __						
TOTAL						
Daily Totals						

Water/Fluid Intake
☐ ☐ ☐ ☐ ☐ ☐ ☐ ☐

Fruits/Vegetables
☐ ☐ ☐ ☐ ☐ ☐ ☐ ☐

Exercise Log

Type	Duration	Calories Burned
TOTAL		

Day/Week	Date	Weight	**159**

Goals for the Day: _____

Morning	Time: __ __:__ __					Mood	Energy
TOTAL							

Afternoon	Time: __ __:__ __						
TOTAL							

Evening	Time: __ __:__ __						
TOTAL							

Snacks							
	Time: __ __:__ __						
	Time: __ __:__ __						
	Time: __ __:__ __						
	Time: __ __:__ __						
TOTAL							
Daily Totals							

Water/Fluid Intake ❑❑❑❑❑❑❑❑   *Fruits/Vegetables* ❑❑❑❑❑❑❑❑

Exercise Log

Type	Duration	Calories Burned
TOTAL		

160

Day/Week	Date	Weight

Goals for the Day: _____

Morning Time: __ __:__ __					Mood	Energy
TOTAL						
Afternoon Time: __ __:__ __						
TOTAL						
Evening Time: __ __:__ __						
TOTAL						
Snacks						
Time: __ __:__ __						
Time: __ __:__ __						
Time: __ __:__ __						
Time: __ __:__ __						
TOTAL						
Daily Totals						

Water/Fluid Intake
❑ ❑ ❑ ❑ ❑ ❑ ❑

Fruits/Vegetables
❑ ❑ ❑ ❑ ❑ ❑ ❑

Exercise Log

Type	Duration	Calories Burned
TOTAL		

Day/Week	Date	Weight

Goals for the Day: _____

Morning	Time: __ __:__ __						Mood	Energy
TOTAL								
Afternoon	Time: __ __:__ __							
TOTAL								
Evening	Time: __ __:__ __							
TOTAL								
Snacks								
	Time: __ __:__ __							
	Time: __ __:__ __							
	Time: __ __:__ __							
	Time: __ __:__ __							
TOTAL								
Daily Totals								

Water/Fluid Intake ❑ ❑ ❑ ❑ ❑ ❑ ❑ ❑   *Fruits/Vegetables* ❑ ❑ ❑ ❑ ❑ ❑ ❑ ❑

Exercise Log

Type	Duration	Calories Burned
TOTAL		

Weekly Assessment

Food Intake Summary

DAY 1				
DAY 2				
DAY 3				
DAY 4				
DAY 5				
DAY 6				
DAY 7				
Weekly Total				
Average Daily Intake (Total ÷ 7)				

Did you meet your goals for water and fruit and veggie intake this week?   Yes   No

Exercise Summary

	Type	Duration	Calories Burned
DAY 1			
DAY 2			
DAY 3			
DAY 4			
DAY 5			
DAY 6			
DAY 7			
TOTALS			

Notes & Gold Star Moments

Goals for Next Week

Eating:

Exercise:

Other:

Day/Week	Date	Weight

Goals for the Day: _____

Morning	Time: __ __:__ __					Mood	Energy
TOTAL							
Afternoon	Time: __ __:__ __						
TOTAL							
Evening	Time: __ __:__ __						
TOTAL							
Snacks							
	Time: __ __:__ __						
	Time: __ __:__ __						
	Time: __ __:__ __						
	Time: __ __:__ __						
TOTAL							
Daily Totals							

Water/Fluid Intake
☐ ☐ ☐ ☐ ☐ ☐ ☐ ☐

Fruits/Vegetables
☐ ☐ ☐ ☐ ☐ ☐ ☐ ☐

Exercise Log

Type	Duration	Calories Burned
TOTAL		

164

Day/Week	Date	Weight

Goals for the Day: _____

Morning	Time: __ __:__ __					Mood	Energy
TOTAL							
Afternoon	Time: __ __:__ __						
TOTAL							
Evening	Time: __ __:__ __						
TOTAL							
Snacks							
	Time: __ __:__ __						
	Time: __ __:__ __						
	Time: __ __:__ __						
	Time: __ __:__ __						
TOTAL							
Daily Totals							

Water/Fluid Intake
☐ ☐ ☐ ☐ ☐ ☐ ☐ ☐

Fruits/Vegetables
☐ ☐ ☐ ☐ ☐ ☐ ☐ ☐

Exercise Log

Type	Duration	Calories Burned
TOTAL		

Goals for the Day: _____

Morning	Time: __ __:__ __					Mood	Energy
TOTAL							
Afternoon	Time: __ __:__ __						
TOTAL							
Evening	Time: __ __:__ __						
TOTAL							
Snacks							
	Time: __ __:__ __						
	Time: __ __:__ __						
	Time: __ __:__ __						
	Time: __ __:__ __						
TOTAL							
Daily Totals							

Water/Fluid Intake
☐ ☐ ☐ ☐ ☐ ☐ ☐ ☐

Fruits/Vegetables
☐ ☐ ☐ ☐ ☐ ☐ ☐ ☐

Exercise Log

Type	Duration	Calories Burned
TOTAL		

166

Day/Week	Date	Weight

Goals for the Day: _____

Morning	Time: __ __:__ __					Mood	Energy
TOTAL							
Afternoon	Time: __ __:__ __						
TOTAL							
Evening	Time: __ __:__ __						
TOTAL							
Snacks							
	Time: __ __:__ __						
	Time: __ __:__ __						
	Time: __ __:__ __						
	Time: __ __:__ __						
TOTAL							
Daily Totals							

Water/Fluid Intake
☐ ☐ ☐ ☐ ☐ ☐ ☐ ☐

Fruits/Vegetables
☐ ☐ ☐ ☐ ☐ ☐ ☐ ☐

Exercise Log

Type	Duration	Calories Burned
TOTAL		

Day/Week	Date	Weight

Goals for the Day: _____

Morning	Time: __ __:__ __						Mood	Energy
TOTAL								
Afternoon	Time: __ __:__ __							
TOTAL								
Evening	Time: __ __:__ __							
TOTAL								
Snacks								
	Time: __ __:__ __							
	Time: __ __:__ __							
	Time: __ __:__ __							
	Time: __ __:__ __							
TOTAL								
Daily Totals								

Water/Fluid Intake
❑ ❑ ❑ ❑ ❑ ❑ ❑ ❑

Fruits/Vegetables
❑ ❑ ❑ ❑ ❑ ❑ ❑ ❑

Exercise Log

Type	Duration	Calories Burned
TOTAL		

168

Goals for the Day: _____

Morning	Time: __ __:__ __					Mood	Energy
TOTAL							
Afternoon	Time: __ __:__ __						
TOTAL							
Evening	Time: __ __:__ __						
TOTAL							
Snacks							
	Time: __ __:__ __						
	Time: __ __:__ __						
	Time: __ __:__ __						
	Time: __ __:__ __						
TOTAL							
Daily Totals							

Water/Fluid Intake
☐ ☐ ☐ ☐ ☐ ☐ ☐ ☐

Fruits/Vegetables
☐ ☐ ☐ ☐ ☐ ☐ ☐

Exercise Log

Type	Duration	Calories Burned
TOTAL		

Day/Week	Date	Weight	*169*

Goals for the Day: _____

Morning	Time: __ __:__ __					Mood	Energy
TOTAL							
Afternoon	Time: __ __:__ __						
TOTAL							
Evening	Time: __ __:__ __						
TOTAL							
Snacks							
	Time: __ __:__ __						
	Time: __ __:__ __						
	Time: __ __:__ __						
	Time: __ __:__ __						
TOTAL							
Daily Totals							

Water/Fluid Intake
☐ ☐ ☐ ☐ ☐ ☐ ☐ ☐

Fruits/Vegetables
☐ ☐ ☐ ☐ ☐ ☐ ☐ ☐

Exercise Log

Type	Duration	Calories Burned
TOTAL		

Weekly Assessment

Food Intake Summary

DAY 1				
DAY 2				
DAY 3				
DAY 4				
DAY 5				
DAY 6				
DAY 7				
Weekly Total				
Average Daily Intake (Total ÷ 7)				

Did you meet your goals for water and fruit and veggie intake this week?   Yes   No

Exercise Summary

	Type	**Duration**	**Calories Burned**
DAY 1			
DAY 2			
DAY 3			
DAY 4			
DAY 5			
DAY 6			
DAY 7			
TOTALS			

Notes & Gold Star Moments

_____
_____
_____
_____
_____
_____
_____
_____
_____
_____
_____
_____
_____
_____

Goals for Next Week

Eating:_____
_____
_____
_____
_____

Exercise:_____
_____
_____

Other:_____
_____

Day/Week	Date	Weight

Goals for the Day: _____

Morning	Time: __ __:__ __					Mood	Energy
TOTAL							
Afternoon	Time: __ __:__ __						
TOTAL							
Evening	Time: __ __:__ __						
TOTAL							
Snacks							
	Time: __ __:__ __						
	Time: __ __:__ __						
	Time: __ __:__ __						
	Time: __ __:__ __						
TOTAL							
Daily Totals							

Water/Fluid Intake
☐ ☐ ☐ ☐ ☐ ☐ ☐ ☐

Fruits/Vegetables
☐ ☐ ☐ ☐ ☐ ☐ ☐ ☐

Exercise Log

Type	Duration	Calories Burned
TOTAL		

172

Goals for the Day: _____

Morning Time: __ __:__ __					Mood	Energy
TOTAL						
Afternoon Time: __ __:__ __						
TOTAL						
Evening Time: __ __:__ __						
TOTAL						
Snacks						
Time: __ __:__ __						
Time: __ __:__ __						
Time: __ __:__ __						
Time: __ __:__ __						
TOTAL						
Daily Totals						

Water/Fluid Intake   *Fruits/Vegetables*
❏ ❏ ❏ ❏ ❏ ❏ ❏ ❏   ❏ ❏ ❏ ❏ ❏ ❏ ❏ ❏

Exercise Log

Type	Duration	Calories Burned
TOTAL		

Day/Week	Date	Weight	**173**

Goals for the Day: _____

Morning	Time: __ __:__ __					Mood	Energy
TOTAL							

Afternoon	Time: __ __:__ __						
TOTAL							

Evening	Time: __ __:__ __						
TOTAL							

Snacks							
Time: __ __:__ __							
Time: __ __:__ __							
Time: __ __:__ __							
Time: __ __:__ __							
TOTAL							

Daily Totals							

Water/Fluid Intake
❑ ❑ ❑ ❑ ❑ ❑ ❑ ❑

Fruits/Vegetables
❑ ❑ ❑ ❑ ❑ ❑ ❑ ❑

Exercise Log

Type	Duration	Calories Burned
TOTAL		

174

Goals for the Day: _____

Morning	Time: __ __:__ __					Mood	Energy
TOTAL							
Afternoon	Time: __ __:__ __						
TOTAL							
Evening	Time: __ __:__ __						
TOTAL							
Snacks							
	Time: __ __:__ __						
	Time: __ __:__ __						
	Time: __ __:__ __						
	Time: __ __:__ __						
TOTAL							
Daily Totals							

Water/Fluid Intake
❑ ❑ ❑ ❑ ❑ ❑ ❑ ❑

Fruits/Vegetables
❑ ❑ ❑ ❑ ❑ ❑ ❑ ❑

Exercise Log

Type	Duration	Calories Burned
TOTAL		

Day/Week	Date	Weight	**175**

Goals for the Day: _____

Morning	Time: __ __:__ __					Mood	Energy
TOTAL							

Afternoon	Time: __ __:__ __						
TOTAL							

Evening	Time: __ __:__ __						
TOTAL							

Snacks							
	Time: __ __:__ __						
	Time: __ __:__ __						
	Time: __ __:__ __						
	Time: __ __:__ __						
TOTAL							
Daily Totals							

Water/Fluid Intake
❏ ❏ ❏ ❏ ❏ ❏ ❏ ❏

Fruits/Vegetables
❏ ❏ ❏ ❏ ❏ ❏ ❏ ❏

Exercise Log

Type	Duration	Calories Burned
TOTAL		

176

Day/Week	Date	Weight

Goals for the Day: _____

Morning	Time: __ __:__ __					Mood	Energy
TOTAL							
Afternoon	Time: __ __:__ __						
TOTAL							
Evening	Time: __ __:__ __						
TOTAL							
Snacks							
	Time: __ __:__ __						
	Time: __ __:__ __						
	Time: __ __:__ __						
	Time: __ __:__ __						
TOTAL							
Daily Totals							

Water/Fluid Intake
❑ ❑ ❑ ❑ ❑ ❑ ❑

Fruits/Vegetables
❑ ❑ ❑ ❑ ❑ ❑ ❑

Exercise Log

Type	Duration	Calories Burned
TOTAL		

Day/Week	Date	Weight

Goals for the Day: _____

Morning	Time: __ __:__ __					Mood	Energy
TOTAL							
Afternoon	Time: __ __:__ __						
TOTAL							
Evening	Time: __ __:__ __						
TOTAL							
Snacks							
	Time: __ __:__ __						
	Time: __ __:__ __						
	Time: __ __:__ __						
	Time: __ __:__ __						
TOTAL							
Daily Totals							

Water/Fluid Intake	Fruits/Vegetables
❑ ❑ ❑ ❑ ❑ ❑ ❑ ❑	❑ ❑ ❑ ❑ ❑ ❑ ❑ ❑

Exercise Log

Type	Duration	Calories Burned
TOTAL		

Weekly Assessment

Food Intake Summary

DAY 1				
DAY 2				
DAY 3				
DAY 4				
DAY 5				
DAY 6				
DAY 7				
Weekly Total				
Average Daily Intake (Total ÷ 7)				

Did you meet your goals for water and fruit and veggie intake this week?   Yes   No

Exercise Summary

	Type	Duration	Calories Burned
DAY 1			
DAY 2			
DAY 3			
DAY 4			
DAY 5			
DAY 6			
DAY 7			
TOTALS			

Notes & Gold Star Moments

_____
_____
_____
_____
_____
_____
_____
_____
_____
_____
_____
_____

Goals for Next Week

Eating: _____
_____
_____
_____
_____

Exercise: _____
_____
_____

Other: _____
_____
_____

Day/Week	Date	Weight

Goals for the Day: _____

Morning	Time: __ __ : __ __					Mood	Energy
	TOTAL						
Afternoon	Time: __ __ : __ __						
	TOTAL						
Evening	Time: __ __ : __ __						
	TOTAL						
Snacks							
	Time: __ __ : __ __						
	Time: __ __ : __ __						
	Time: __ __ : __ __						
	Time: __ __ : __ __						
	TOTAL						
Daily Totals							

Water/Fluid Intake
❑ ❑ ❑ ❑ ❑ ❑ ❑ ❑

Fruits/Vegetables
❑ ❑ ❑ ❑ ❑ ❑ ❑ ❑

Exercise Log

Type	Duration	Calories Burned
TOTAL		

180

Day/Week	Date	Weight

Goals for the Day: _____

Morning	Time: __ __:__ __					Mood	Energy
TOTAL							
Afternoon	Time: __ __:__ __						
TOTAL							
Evening	Time: __ __:__ __						
TOTAL							
Snacks							
	Time: __ __:__ __						
	Time: __ __:__ __						
	Time: __ __:__ __						
	Time: __ __:__ __						
TOTAL							
Daily Totals							

Water/Fluid Intake
❑ ❑ ❑ ❑ ❑ ❑ ❑ ❑

Fruits/Vegetables
❑ ❑ ❑ ❑ ❑ ❑ ❑ ❑

Exercise Log

Type	Duration	Calories Burned
TOTAL		

Goals for the Day: _____

Morning	Time: __ __:__ __					Mood	Energy
TOTAL							
Afternoon	Time: __ __:__ __						
TOTAL							
Evening	Time: __ __:__ __						
TOTAL							
Snacks							
	Time: __ __:__ __						
	Time: __ __:__ __						
	Time: __ __:__ __						
	Time: __ __:__ __						
TOTAL							
Daily Totals							

Water/Fluid Intake
❑ ❑ ❑ ❑ ❑ ❑ ❑ ❑

Fruits/Vegetables
❑ ❑ ❑ ❑ ❑ ❑ ❑ ❑

Exercise Log

Type	Duration	Calories Burned
TOTAL		

182

Day/Week	Date	Weight

Goals for the Day: _____

Morning	Time: __ __:__ __						Mood	Energy
TOTAL								
Afternoon	Time: __ __:__ __							
TOTAL								
Evening	Time: __ __:__ __							
TOTAL								
Snacks								
	Time: __ __:__ __							
	Time: __ __:__ __							
	Time: __ __:__ __							
	Time: __ __:__ __							
TOTAL								
Daily Totals								

Water/Fluid Intake
❏ ❏ ❏ ❏ ❏ ❏ ❏ ❏

Fruits/Vegetables
❏ ❏ ❏ ❏ ❏ ❏ ❏ ❏

Exercise Log

Type	Duration	Calories Burned
TOTAL		

Goals for the Day: _____

Morning	Time: __ __:__ __					Mood	Energy
TOTAL							
Afternoon	Time: __ __:__ __						
TOTAL							
Evening	Time: __ __:__ __						
TOTAL							
Snacks							
	Time: __ __:__ __						
	Time: __ __:__ __						
	Time: __ __:__ __						
	Time: __ __:__ __						
TOTAL							
Daily Totals							

Water/Fluid Intake
❑❑❑❑❑❑❑❑

Fruits/Vegetables
❑❑❑❑❑❑❑❑

Exercise Log

Type	Duration	Calories Burned
TOTAL		

184

Goals for the Day: _____

Morning	Time: __ __:__ __						Mood	Energy
TOTAL								
Afternoon	Time: __ __:__ __							
TOTAL								
Evening	Time: __ __:__ __							
TOTAL								
Snacks								
	Time: __ __:__ __							
	Time: __ __:__ __							
	Time: __ __:__ __							
	Time: __ __:__ __							
TOTAL								
Daily Totals								

Water/Fluid Intake
▢ ▢ ▢ ▢ ▢ ▢ ▢ ▢

Fruits/Vegetables
▢ ▢ ▢ ▢ ▢ ▢ ▢ ▢

Exercise Log

Type	Duration	Calories Burned
TOTAL		

Day/Week	Date	Weight	*185*

Goals for the Day: _____

Morning	Time: __ __:__ __					Mood	Energy
TOTAL							
Afternoon	Time: __ __:__ __						
TOTAL							
Evening	Time: __ __:__ __						
TOTAL							
Snacks							
	Time: __ __:__ __						
	Time: __ __:__ __						
	Time: __ __:__ __						
	Time: __ __:__ __						
TOTAL							
Daily Totals							

Water/Fluid Intake
❑ ❑ ❑ ❑ ❑ ❑ ❑ ❑

Fruits/Vegetables
❑ ❑ ❑ ❑ ❑ ❑ ❑ ❑

Exercise Log

Type	Duration	Calories Burned
TOTAL		

Weekly Assessment

Food Intake Summary

DAY 1				
DAY 2				
DAY 3				
DAY 4				
DAY 5				
DAY 6				
DAY 7				
Weekly Total				
Average Daily Intake (Total ÷ 7)				

Did you meet your goals for water and fruit and veggie intake this week?　　Yes　No

Exercise Summary

	Type	Duration	Calories Burned
DAY 1			
DAY 2			
DAY 3			
DAY 4			
DAY 5			
DAY 6			
DAY 7			
TOTALS			

Notes & Gold Star Moments

_____
_____
_____
_____
_____
_____
_____
_____
_____
_____

Goals for Next Week

Eating: _____
_____
_____
_____

Exercise: _____
_____
_____

Other: _____
_____

Day/Week	Date	Weight

Goals for the Day: _____

Morning	Time: __ __:__ __					Mood	Energy
TOTAL							

Afternoon	Time: __ __:__ __						
TOTAL							

Evening	Time: __ __:__ __						
TOTAL							

Snacks							
	Time: __ __:__ __						
	Time: __ __:__ __						
	Time: __ __:__ __						
	Time: __ __:__ __						
TOTAL							
Daily Totals							

Water/Fluid Intake ❑ ❑ ❑ ❑ ❑ ❑ ❑ ❑   **Fruits/Vegetables** ❑ ❑ ❑ ❑ ❑ ❑ ❑ ❑

Exercise Log

Type	Duration	Calories Burned
TOTAL		

Day/Week	Date	Weight

Goals for the Day: _____

Morning	Time: __ __:__ __					Mood	Energy
TOTAL							

Afternoon	Time: __ __:__ __						
TOTAL							

Evening	Time: __ __:__ __						
TOTAL							

Snacks							
	Time: __ __:__ __						
	Time: __ __:__ __						
	Time: __ __:__ __						
	Time: __ __:__ __						
TOTAL							
Daily Totals							

Water/Fluid Intake
☐ ☐ ☐ ☐ ☐ ☐ ☐ ☐

Fruits/Vegetables
☐ ☐ ☐ ☐ ☐ ☐ ☐ ☐

Exercise Log

Type	Duration	Calories Burned
TOTAL		

Day/Week	Date	Weight

Goals for the Day: _____

Morning	Time: __ __:__ __					Mood	Energy
TOTAL							
Afternoon	Time: __ __:__ __						
TOTAL							
Evening	Time: __ __:__ __						
TOTAL							
Snacks							
	Time: __ __:__ __						
	Time: __ __:__ __						
	Time: __ __:__ __						
	Time: __ __:__ __						
TOTAL							
Daily Totals							

Water/Fluid Intake
❏ ❏ ❏ ❏ ❏ ❏ ❏ ❏

Fruits/Vegetables
❏ ❏ ❏ ❏ ❏ ❏ ❏ ❏

Exercise Log

Type	Duration	Calories Burned
TOTAL		

190

Day/Week	Date	Weight

Goals for the Day: _____

Morning	Time: __ __:__ __					Mood	Energy
TOTAL							
Afternoon	Time: __ __:__ __						
TOTAL							
Evening	Time: __ __:__ __						
TOTAL							
Snacks							
	Time: __ __:__ __						
	Time: __ __:__ __						
	Time: __ __:__ __						
	Time: __ __:__ __						
TOTAL							
Daily Totals							

Water/Fluid Intake
❏ ❏ ❏ ❏ ❏ ❏ ❏ ❏

Fruits/Vegetables
❏ ❏ ❏ ❏ ❏ ❏ ❏ ❏

Exercise Log

Type	Duration	Calories Burned
TOTAL		

Day/Week	Date	Weight	

191

Goals for the Day: _____

Morning	Time: __ __:__ __						Mood	Energy
TOTAL								
Afternoon	Time: __ __:__ __							
TOTAL								
Evening	Time: __ __:__ __							
TOTAL								
Snacks								
	Time: __ __:__ __							
	Time: __ __:__ __							
	Time: __ __:__ __							
	Time: __ __:__ __							
TOTAL								
Daily Totals								

Water/Fluid Intake
❑ ❑ ❑ ❑ ❑ ❑ ❑ ❑

Fruits/Vegetables
❑ ❑ ❑ ❑ ❑ ❑ ❑ ❑

Exercise Log

Type	Duration	Calories Burned
TOTAL		

192

Goals for the Day: _____

Morning	Time: __ __:__ __					Mood	Energy
TOTAL							
Afternoon	Time: __ __:__ __						
TOTAL							
Evening	Time: __ __:__ __						
TOTAL							
Snacks							
	Time: __ __:__ __						
	Time: __ __:__ __						
	Time: __ __:__ __						
	Time: __ __:__ __						
TOTAL							
Daily Totals							

Water/Fluid Intake
❑ ❑ ❑ ❑ ❑ ❑ ❑ ❑

Fruits/Vegetables
❑ ❑ ❑ ❑ ❑ ❑ ❑ ❑

Exercise Log

Type	Duration	Calories Burned
TOTAL		

Day/Week	Date	Weight	*193*

Goals for the Day: _____

Morning Time: __ __:__ __					Mood	Energy
TOTAL						
Afternoon Time: __ __:__ __						
TOTAL						
Evening Time: __ __:__ __						
TOTAL						
Snacks						
Time: __ __:__ __						
Time: __ __:__ __						
Time: __ __:__ __						
Time: __ __:__ __						
TOTAL						
Daily Totals						

Water/Fluid Intake
❏ ❏ ❏ ❏ ❏ ❏ ❏

Fruits/Vegetables
❏ ❏ ❏ ❏ ❏ ❏ ❏

Exercise Log

Type	Duration	Calories Burned
TOTAL		

Weekly Assessment

Food Intake Summary

DAY 1				
DAY 2				
DAY 3				
DAY 4				
DAY 5				
DAY 6				
DAY 7				
Weekly Total				
Average Daily Intake (Total ÷ 7)				

Did you meet your goals for water and fruit and veggie intake this week?   Yes   No

Exercise Summary

	Type	Duration	Calories Burned
DAY 1			
DAY 2			
DAY 3			
DAY 4			
DAY 5			
DAY 6			
DAY 7			
TOTALS			

Notes & Gold Star Moments

_____
_____
_____
_____
_____
_____
_____
_____
_____
_____
_____

Goals for Next Week

Eating: _____
_____
_____
_____
_____

Exercise: _____
_____
_____

Other: _____

Day/Week	Date	Weight

Goals for the Day: _____

Morning	Time: __ __:__ __						Mood	Energy
TOTAL								
Afternoon	Time: __ __:__ __							
TOTAL								
Evening	Time: __ __:__ __							
TOTAL								
Snacks								
	Time: __ __:__ __							
	Time: __ __:__ __							
	Time: __ __:__ __							
	Time: __ __:__ __							
TOTAL								
Daily Totals								

Water/Fluid Intake
❏ ❏ ❏ ❏ ❏ ❏ ❏ ❏

Fruits/Vegetables
❏ ❏ ❏ ❏ ❏ ❏ ❏ ❏

Exercise Log

Type	Duration	Calories Burned
TOTAL		

196

Day/Week	Date	Weight

Goals for the Day: _____

Morning	Time: __ __:__ __						Mood	Energy
TOTAL								
Afternoon	Time: __ __:__ __							
TOTAL								
Evening	Time: __ __:__ __							
TOTAL								
Snacks								
	Time: __ __:__ __							
	Time: __ __:__ __							
	Time: __ __:__ __							
	Time: __ __:__ __							
TOTAL								
Daily Totals								

Water/Fluid Intake
❏ ❏ ❏ ❏ ❏ ❏ ❏ ❏

Fruits/Vegetables
❏ ❏ ❏ ❏ ❏ ❏ ❏ ❏

Exercise Log

Type	Duration	Calories Burned
TOTAL		

Day/Week	Date	Weight

Goals for the Day: _____

Morning	Time: __ __:__ __					Mood	Energy
TOTAL							
Afternoon	Time: __ __:__ __						
TOTAL							
Evening	Time: __ __:__ __						
TOTAL							
Snacks							
	Time: __ __:__ __						
	Time: __ __:__ __						
	Time: __ __:__ __						
	Time: __ __:__ __						
TOTAL							
Daily Totals							

Water/Fluid Intake
☐ ☐ ☐ ☐ ☐ ☐ ☐ ☐

Fruits/Vegetables
☐ ☐ ☐ ☐ ☐ ☐ ☐ ☐

Exercise Log

Type	Duration	Calories Burned
TOTAL		

198

Goals for the Day: _____

Morning	Time: __ __:__ __					Mood	Energy
TOTAL							

Afternoon	Time: __ __:__ __						
TOTAL							

Evening	Time: __ __:__ __						
TOTAL							

Snacks							
	Time: __ __:__ __						
	Time: __ __:__ __						
	Time: __ __:__ __						
	Time: __ __:__ __						
TOTAL							
Daily Totals							

Water/Fluid Intake
☐ ☐ ☐ ☐ ☐ ☐ ☐ ☐

Fruits/Vegetables
☐ ☐ ☐ ☐ ☐ ☐ ☐ ☐

Exercise Log

Type	Duration	Calories Burned
TOTAL		

Day/Week	Date	Weight

Goals for the Day: _____

Morning	Time: __ __:__ __					Mood	Energy
TOTAL							
Afternoon	Time: __ __:__ __						
TOTAL							
Evening	Time: __ __:__ __						
TOTAL							
Snacks							
	Time: __ __:__ __						
	Time: __ __:__ __						
	Time: __ __:__ __						
	Time: __ __:__ __						
TOTAL							
Daily Totals							

Water/Fluid Intake
☐ ☐ ☐ ☐ ☐ ☐ ☐ ☐

Fruits/Vegetables
☐ ☐ ☐ ☐ ☐ ☐ ☐ ☐

Exercise Log

Type	Duration	Calories Burned
TOTAL		

Day/Week	Date	Weight

Goals for the Day: _____

Morning Time: __ __:__ __						Mood	Energy
TOTAL							
Afternoon Time: __ __:__ __							
TOTAL							
Evening Time: __ __:__ __							
TOTAL							
Snacks							
Time: __ __:__ __							
Time: __ __:__ __							
Time: __ __:__ __							
Time: __ __:__ __							
TOTAL							
Daily Totals							

Water/Fluid Intake
☐ ☐ ☐ ☐ ☐ ☐ ☐ ☐

Fruits/Vegetables
☐ ☐ ☐ ☐ ☐ ☐ ☐ ☐

Exercise Log

Type	Duration	Calories Burned
TOTAL		

| Day/Week | Date | Weight | *201* |

Goals for the Day: _____

Morning	Time: __ __:__ __						Mood	Energy
TOTAL								
Afternoon	Time: __ __:__ __							
TOTAL								
Evening	Time: __ __:__ __							
TOTAL								
Snacks								
	Time: __ __:__ __							
	Time: __ __:__ __							
	Time: __ __:__ __							
	Time: __ __:__ __							
TOTAL								
Daily Totals								

Water/Fluid Intake
□ □ □ □ □ □ □ □

Fruits/Vegetables
□ □ □ □ □ □ □ □

Exercise Log

Type	Duration	Calories Burned
TOTAL		

202 *Weekly Assessment*

Food Intake Summary

DAY 1				
DAY 2				
DAY 3				
DAY 4				
DAY 5				
DAY 6				
DAY 7				
Weekly Total				
Average Daily Intake (Total ÷ 7)				

Did you meet your goals for water and fruit and veggie intake this week?   Yes   No

Exercise Summary

	Type	Duration	Calories Burned
DAY 1			
DAY 2			
DAY 3			
DAY 4			
DAY 5			
DAY 6			
DAY 7			
TOTALS			

Notes & Gold Star Moments

Goals for Next Week

Eating:

Exercise:

Other:

Day/Week	Date	Weight	**203**

Goals for the Day: _____

Morning	Time: __ __:__ __					Mood	Energy
TOTAL							

Afternoon	Time: __ __:__ __						
TOTAL							

Evening	Time: __ __:__ __						
TOTAL							

Snacks							
	Time: __ __:__ __						
	Time: __ __:__ __						
	Time: __ __:__ __						
	Time: __ __:__ __						
TOTAL							

Daily Totals							

Water/Fluid Intake
☐ ☐ ☐ ☐ ☐ ☐ ☐ ☐

Fruits/Vegetables
☐ ☐ ☐ ☐ ☐ ☐ ☐ ☐

Exercise Log

Type	Duration	Calories Burned
TOTAL		

204

Day/Week	Date	Weight

Goals for the Day: _____

Morning	Time: __ __:__ __						Mood	Energy
TOTAL								
Afternoon	Time: __ __:__ __							
TOTAL								
Evening	Time: __ __:__ __							
TOTAL								
Snacks								
	Time: __ __:__ __							
	Time: __ __:__ __							
	Time: __ __:__ __							
	Time: __ __:__ __							
TOTAL								
Daily Totals								

Water/Fluid Intake
☐ ☐ ☐ ☐ ☐ ☐ ☐

Fruits/Vegetables
☐ ☐ ☐ ☐ ☐ ☐ ☐ ☐

Exercise Log

Type	Duration	Calories Burned
TOTAL		

Day/Week	Date	Weight

Goals for the Day: _____

Morning	Time: __ __:__ __					Mood	Energy
TOTAL							
Afternoon	Time: __ __:__ __						
TOTAL							
Evening	Time: __ __:__ __						
TOTAL							
Snacks							
	Time: __ __:__ __						
	Time: __ __:__ __						
	Time: __ __:__ __						
	Time: __ __:__ __						
TOTAL							
Daily Totals							

Water/Fluid Intake
☐ ☐ ☐ ☐ ☐ ☐ ☐ ☐

Fruits/Vegetables
☐ ☐ ☐ ☐ ☐ ☐ ☐ ☐

Exercise Log

Type	Duration	Calories Burned
TOTAL		

206

Goals for the Day: _____

Morning Time: __ __:__ __					Mood	Energy
TOTAL						
Afternoon Time: __ __:__ __						
TOTAL						
Evening Time: __ __:__ __						
TOTAL						
Snacks						
Time: __ __:__ __						
Time: __ __:__ __						
Time: __ __:__ __						
Time: __ __:__ __						
TOTAL						
Daily Totals						

Water/Fluid Intake
❑ ❑ ❑ ❑ ❑ ❑ ❑ ❑

Fruits/Vegetables
❑ ❑ ❑ ❑ ❑ ❑ ❑ ❑

Exercise Log

Type	Duration	Calories Burned
TOTAL		

Day/Week	Date	Weight

Goals for the Day: _____

Morning Time: __ __:__ __						Mood	Energy
TOTAL							
Afternoon Time: __ __:__ __							
TOTAL							
Evening Time: __ __:__ __							
TOTAL							
Snacks							
Time: __ __:__ __							
Time: __ __:__ __							
Time: __ __:__ __							
Time: __ __:__ __							
TOTAL							
Daily Totals							

Water/Fluid Intake
☐ ☐ ☐ ☐ ☐ ☐ ☐ ☐

Fruits/Vegetables
☐ ☐ ☐ ☐ ☐ ☐ ☐ ☐

Exercise Log

Type	Duration	Calories Burned
TOTAL		

208

Day/Week	Date	Weight

Goals for the Day: _____

Morning	Time: __ __:__ __					Mood	Energy
TOTAL							
Afternoon	Time: __ __:__ __						
TOTAL							
Evening	Time: __ __:__ __						
TOTAL							
Snacks							
	Time: __ __:__ __						
	Time: __ __:__ __						
	Time: __ __:__ __						
	Time: __ __:__ __						
TOTAL							
Daily Totals							

Water/Fluid Intake
❑ ❑ ❑ ❑ ❑ ❑ ❑ ❑

Fruits/Vegetables
❑ ❑ ❑ ❑ ❑ ❑ ❑ ❑

Exercise Log

Type	Duration	Calories Burned
TOTAL		

Day/Week	Date	Weight

Goals for the Day: _____

Morning	Time: __ __:__ __						Mood	Energy
TOTAL								
Afternoon	Time: __ __:__ __							
TOTAL								
Evening	Time: __ __:__ __							
TOTAL								
Snacks								
	Time: __ __:__ __							
	Time: __ __:__ __							
	Time: __ __:__ __							
	Time: __ __:__ __							
TOTAL								
Daily Totals								

Water/Fluid Intake
❑❑❑❑❑❑❑❑

Fruits/Vegetables
❑❑❑❑❑❑❑❑

Exercise Log

Type	Duration	Calories Burned
TOTAL		

Weekly Assessment

Food Intake Summary

DAY 1				
DAY 2				
DAY 3				
DAY 4				
DAY 5				
DAY 6				
DAY 7				
Weekly Total				
Average Daily Intake (Total ÷ 7)				

Did you meet your goals for water and fruit and veggie intake this week?   Yes   No

Exercise Summary

	Type	Duration	Calories Burned
DAY 1			
DAY 2			
DAY 3			
DAY 4			
DAY 5			
DAY 6			
DAY 7			
TOTALS			

Notes & Gold Star Moments

_____
_____
_____
_____
_____
_____
_____
_____
_____
_____
_____

Goals for Next Week

Eating: _____
_____
_____
_____
_____

Exercise: _____
_____
_____

Other: _____
_____

Day/Week	Date	Weight

Goals for the Day: _____

Morning	Time: __ __:__ __					Mood	Energy
TOTAL							
Afternoon	Time: __ __:__ __						
TOTAL							
Evening	Time: __ __:__ __						
TOTAL							
Snacks							
	Time: __ __:__ __						
	Time: __ __:__ __						
	Time: __ __:__ __						
	Time: __ __:__ __						
TOTAL							
Daily Totals							

Water/Fluid Intake
❑ ❑ ❑ ❑ ❑ ❑ ❑ ❑

Fruits/Vegetables
❑ ❑ ❑ ❑ ❑ ❑ ❑ ❑

Exercise Log

Type	Duration	Calories Burned
TOTAL		

212

Day/Week	Date	Weight

Goals for the Day: _____

Morning	Time: __ __:__ __						Mood	Energy
TOTAL								
Afternoon	Time: __ __:__ __							
TOTAL								
Evening	Time: __ __:__ __							
TOTAL								
Snacks								
	Time: __ __:__ __							
	Time: __ __:__ __							
	Time: __ __:__ __							
	Time: __ __:__ __							
TOTAL								
Daily Totals								

Water/Fluid Intake
❑ ❑ ❑ ❑ ❑ ❑ ❑

Fruits/Vegetables
❑ ❑ ❑ ❑ ❑ ❑ ❑

Exercise Log

Type	Duration	Calories Burned
TOTAL		

Day/Week	Date	Weight	**213**

Goals for the Day: _____

Morning	Time: __ __:__ __					Mood	Energy
TOTAL							
Afternoon	Time: __ __:__ __						
TOTAL							
Evening	Time: __ __:__ __						
TOTAL							
Snacks							
	Time: __ __:__ __						
	Time: __ __:__ __						
	Time: __ __:__ __						
	Time: __ __:__ __						
TOTAL							
Daily Totals							

Water/Fluid Intake ❑❑❑❑❑❑❑❑   **Fruits/Vegetables** ❑❑❑❑❑❑❑❑

Exercise Log

Type	Duration	Calories Burned
TOTAL		

214

Day/Week	Date	Weight

Goals for the Day: _____

Morning	Time: __ __:__ __						Mood	Energy
TOTAL								
Afternoon	Time: __ __:__ __							
TOTAL								
Evening	Time: __ __:__ __							
TOTAL								
Snacks								
	Time: __ __:__ __							
	Time: __ __:__ __							
	Time: __ __:__ __							
	Time: __ __:__ __							
TOTAL								
Daily Totals								

Water/Fluid Intake
❑ ❑ ❑ ❑ ❑ ❑ ❑ ❑

Fruits/Vegetables
❑ ❑ ❑ ❑ ❑ ❑ ❑ ❑

Exercise Log

Type	Duration	Calories Burned
TOTAL		

Day/Week	Date	Weight

Goals for the Day: _____

Morning	Time: __ __:__ __					Mood	Energy
TOTAL							

Afternoon	Time: __ __:__ __						
TOTAL							

Evening	Time: __ __:__ __						
TOTAL							

Snacks							
Time: __ __:__ __							
Time: __ __:__ __							
Time: __ __:__ __							
Time: __ __:__ __							
TOTAL							

Daily Totals							

Water/Fluid Intake
☐ ☐ ☐ ☐ ☐ ☐ ☐ ☐

Fruits/Vegetables
☐ ☐ ☐ ☐ ☐ ☐ ☐ ☐

Exercise Log

Type	Duration	Calories Burned
TOTAL		

216

Goals for the Day: _____

Morning	Time: __ __:__ __					Mood	Energy
TOTAL							
Afternoon	Time: __ __:__ __						
TOTAL							
Evening	Time: __ __:__ __						
TOTAL							
Snacks							
	Time: __ __:__ __						
	Time: __ __:__ __						
	Time: __ __:__ __						
	Time: __ __:__ __						
TOTAL							
Daily Totals							

Water/Fluid Intake
☐ ☐ ☐ ☐ ☐ ☐ ☐ ☐

Fruits/Vegetables
☐ ☐ ☐ ☐ ☐ ☐ ☐ ☐

Exercise Log

Type	Duration	Calories Burned
TOTAL		

| Day/Week | Date | Weight | **217** |

Goals for the Day: _____

Morning	Time: __ __:__ __					Mood	Energy
TOTAL							
Afternoon	Time: __ __:__ __						
TOTAL							
Evening	Time: __ __:__ __						
TOTAL							
Snacks							
	Time: __ __:__ __						
	Time: __ __:__ __						
	Time: __ __:__ __						
	Time: __ __:__ __						
TOTAL							
Daily Totals							

Water/Fluid Intake
☐ ☐ ☐ ☐ ☐ ☐ ☐ ☐

Fruits/Vegetables
☐ ☐ ☐ ☐ ☐ ☐ ☐ ☐

Exercise Log

Type	Duration	Calories Burned
TOTAL		

Weekly Assessment

Food Intake Summary

DAY 1				
DAY 2				
DAY 3				
DAY 4				
DAY 5				
DAY 6				
DAY 7				
Weekly Total				
Average Daily Intake (Total ÷ 7)				

Did you meet your goals for water and fruit and veggie intake this week?   Yes   No

Exercise Summary

	Type	Duration	Calories Burned
DAY 1			
DAY 2			
DAY 3			
DAY 4			
DAY 5			
DAY 6			
DAY 7			
TOTALS			

Notes & Gold Star Moments

Goals for Next Week

Eating: _____

Exercise: _____

Other: _____

Day/Week	Date	Weight

Goals for the Day: _____

Morning	Time: __ __:__ __					Mood	Energy
TOTAL							
Afternoon	Time: __ __:__ __						
TOTAL							
Evening	Time: __ __:__ __						
TOTAL							
Snacks							
	Time: __ __:__ __						
	Time: __ __:__ __						
	Time: __ __:__ __						
	Time: __ __:__ __						
TOTAL							
Daily Totals							

Water/Fluid Intake
☐ ☐ ☐ ☐ ☐ ☐ ☐ ☐

Fruits/Vegetables
☐ ☐ ☐ ☐ ☐ ☐ ☐ ☐

Exercise Log

Type	Duration	Calories Burned
TOTAL		

220

Goals for the Day: _____

Morning	Time: __ __:__ __					Mood	Energy
TOTAL							
Afternoon	Time: __ __:__ __						
TOTAL							
Evening	Time: __ __:__ __						
TOTAL							
Snacks							
	Time: __ __:__ __						
	Time: __ __:__ __						
	Time: __ __:__ __						
	Time: __ __:__ __						
TOTAL							
Daily Totals							

Water/Fluid Intake
❑ ❑ ❑ ❑ ❑ ❑ ❑ ❑

Fruits/Vegetables
❑ ❑ ❑ ❑ ❑ ❑ ❑ ❑

Exercise Log

Type	Duration	Calories Burned
TOTAL		

Day/Week	Date	Weight	**221**

Goals for the Day: _____

Morning	Time: __ __:__ __						Mood	Energy
TOTAL								
Afternoon	Time: __ __:__ __							
TOTAL								
Evening	Time: __ __:__ __							
TOTAL								
Snacks								
	Time: __ __:__ __							
	Time: __ __:__ __							
	Time: __ __:__ __							
	Time: __ __:__ __							
TOTAL								
Daily Totals								

Water/Fluid Intake
❏ ❏ ❏ ❏ ❏ ❏ ❏ ❏

Fruits/Vegetables
❏ ❏ ❏ ❏ ❏ ❏ ❏ ❏

Exercise Log

Type	Duration	Calories Burned
TOTAL		

Day/Week	Date	Weight

Goals for the Day: _____

Morning	Time: __ __ : __ __					Mood	Energy
TOTAL							

Afternoon	Time: __ __ : __ __						
TOTAL							

Evening	Time: __ __ : __ __						
TOTAL							

Snacks							
Time: __ __ : __ __							
Time: __ __ : __ __							
Time: __ __ : __ __							
Time: __ __ : __ __							
TOTAL							
Daily Totals							

Water/Fluid Intake
❑ ❑ ❑ ❑ ❑ ❑ ❑ ❑

Fruits/Vegetables
❑ ❑ ❑ ❑ ❑ ❑ ❑ ❑

Exercise Log

Type	Duration	Calories Burned
TOTAL		

Day/Week	Date	Weight	**223**

Goals for the Day: _____

Morning	Time: __ __:__ __						Mood	Energy
TOTAL								
Afternoon	Time: __ __:__ __							
TOTAL								
Evening	Time: __ __:__ __							
TOTAL								
Snacks								
	Time: __ __:__ __							
	Time: __ __:__ __							
	Time: __ __:__ __							
	Time: __ __:__ __							
TOTAL								
Daily Totals								

Water/Fluid Intake
☐ ☐ ☐ ☐ ☐ ☐ ☐ ☐

Fruits/Vegetables
☐ ☐ ☐ ☐ ☐ ☐ ☐ ☐

Exercise Log

Type	Duration	Calories Burned
TOTAL		

224

Day/Week	Date	Weight

Goals for the Day: _____

Morning	Time: __ __:__ __					Mood	Energy
TOTAL							
Afternoon	Time: __ __:__ __						
TOTAL							
Evening	Time: __ __:__ __						
TOTAL							
Snacks							
	Time: __ __:__ __						
	Time: __ __:__ __						
	Time: __ __:__ __						
	Time: __ __:__ __						
TOTAL							
Daily Totals							

Water/Fluid Intake
❑ ❑ ❑ ❑ ❑ ❑ ❑ ❑

Fruits/Vegetables
❑ ❑ ❑ ❑ ❑ ❑ ❑ ❑

Exercise Log

Type	Duration	Calories Burned
TOTAL		

Day/Week	Date	Weight	*225*

Goals for the Day: _____

Morning	Time: __ __:__ __						Mood	Energy
TOTAL								

Afternoon	Time: __ __:__ __							
TOTAL								

Evening	Time: __ __:__ __							
TOTAL								

Snacks								
	Time: __ __:__ __							
	Time: __ __:__ __							
	Time: __ __:__ __							
	Time: __ __:__ __							
TOTAL								
Daily Totals								

Water/Fluid Intake
❑ ❑ ❑ ❑ ❑ ❑ ❑ ❑

Fruits/Vegetables
❑ ❑ ❑ ❑ ❑ ❑ ❑

Exercise Log

Type	Duration	Calories Burned
TOTAL		

Food Intake Summary

DAY 1				
DAY 2				
DAY 3				
DAY 4				
DAY 5				
DAY 6				
DAY 7				
Weekly Total				
Average Daily Intake (Total ÷ 7)				

Did you meet your goals for water and fruit and veggie intake this week?   Yes   No

Exercise Summary

	Type	Duration	Calories Burned
DAY 1			
DAY 2			
DAY 3			
DAY 4			
DAY 5			
DAY 6			
DAY 7			
TOTALS			

Notes & Gold Star Moments

_____
_____
_____
_____
_____
_____
_____
_____
_____
_____
_____
_____

Goals for Next Week

Eating: _____
_____
_____
_____
_____

Exercise: _____
_____
_____

Other: _____
_____

Day/Week	Date	Weight

Goals for the Day: _____

Morning	Time: __ __:__ __					Mood	Energy
TOTAL							
Afternoon	Time: __ __:__ __						
TOTAL							
Evening	Time: __ __:__ __						
TOTAL							
Snacks							
	Time: __ __:__ __						
	Time: __ __:__ __						
	Time: __ __:__ __						
	Time: __ __:__ __						
TOTAL							
Daily Totals							

Water/Fluid Intake
☐ ☐ ☐ ☐ ☐ ☐ ☐ ☐

Fruits/Vegetables
☐ ☐ ☐ ☐ ☐ ☐ ☐ ☐

Exercise Log

Type	Duration	Calories Burned
TOTAL		

228

Day/Week	Date	Weight

Goals for the Day: _____

Morning	Time: __ __:__ __					Mood	Energy
TOTAL							
Afternoon	Time: __ __:__ __						
TOTAL							
Evening	Time: __ __:__ __						
TOTAL							
Snacks							
	Time: __ __:__ __						
	Time: __ __:__ __						
	Time: __ __:__ __						
	Time: __ __:__ __						
TOTAL							
Daily Totals							

Water/Fluid Intake   *Fruits/Vegetables*
☐ ☐ ☐ ☐ ☐ ☐ ☐   ☐ ☐ ☐ ☐ ☐ ☐ ☐ ☐

Exercise Log

Type	Duration	Calories Burned
TOTAL		

Day/Week	Date	Weight	**229**

Goals for the Day: _____

Morning	Time: __ __:__ __						Mood	Energy
TOTAL								
Afternoon	Time: __ __:__ __							
TOTAL								
Evening	Time: __ __:__ __							
TOTAL								
Snacks								
	Time: __ __:__ __							
	Time: __ __:__ __							
	Time: __ __:__ __							
	Time: __ __:__ __							
TOTAL								
Daily Totals								

Water/Fluid Intake
❑ ❑ ❑ ❑ ❑ ❑ ❑ ❑

Fruits/Vegetables
❑ ❑ ❑ ❑ ❑ ❑ ❑ ❑

Exercise Log

Type	Duration	Calories Burned
TOTAL		

Day/Week	Date	Weight

Goals for the Day: _____

Morning	Time: __ __:__ __						Mood	Energy
TOTAL								
Afternoon	Time: __ __:__ __							
TOTAL								
Evening	Time: __ __:__ __							
TOTAL								
Snacks								
	Time: __ __:__ __							
	Time: __ __:__ __							
	Time: __ __:__ __							
	Time: __ __:__ __							
TOTAL								
Daily Totals								

Water/Fluid Intake
❏ ❏ ❏ ❏ ❏ ❏ ❏ ❏

Fruits/Vegetables
❏ ❏ ❏ ❏ ❏ ❏ ❏ ❏

Exercise Log

Type	Duration	Calories Burned
TOTAL		

Day/Week	Date	Weight	**231**

Goals for the Day: _____

Morning	Time: __ __:__ __						Mood	Energy
TOTAL								
Afternoon	Time: __ __:__ __							
TOTAL								
Evening	Time: __ __:__ __							
TOTAL								
Snacks								
	Time: __ __:__ __							
	Time: __ __:__ __							
	Time: __ __:__ __							
	Time: __ __:__ __							
TOTAL								
Daily Totals								

Water/Fluid Intake
❑ ❑ ❑ ❑ ❑ ❑ ❑ ❑

Fruits/Vegetables
❑ ❑ ❑ ❑ ❑ ❑ ❑ ❑

Exercise Log

Type	Duration	Calories Burned
TOTAL		

Day/Week	Date	Weight

Goals for the Day: _____

Morning Time: __ __:__ __					Mood	Energy
TOTAL						
Afternoon Time: __ __:__ __						
TOTAL						
Evening Time: __ __:__ __						
TOTAL						
Snacks						
Time: __ __:__ __						
Time: __ __:__ __						
Time: __ __:__ __						
Time: __ __:__ __						
TOTAL						
Daily Totals						

Water/Fluid Intake
❑ ❑ ❑ ❑ ❑ ❑ ❑

Fruits/Vegetables
❑ ❑ ❑ ❑ ❑ ❑ ❑

Exercise Log

Type	Duration	Calories Burned
TOTAL		

Day/Week	Date	Weight	233

Goals for the Day: _____

Morning	Time: __ __:__ __						Mood	Energy
TOTAL								
Afternoon	Time: __ __:__ __							
TOTAL								
Evening	Time: __ __:__ __							
TOTAL								
Snacks								
	Time: __ __:__ __							
	Time: __ __:__ __							
	Time: __ __:__ __							
	Time: __ __:__ __							
TOTAL								
Daily Totals								

Water/Fluid Intake
❑ ❑ ❑ ❑ ❑ ❑ ❑ ❑

Fruits/Vegetables
❑ ❑ ❑ ❑ ❑ ❑ ❑ ❑

Exercise Log

Type	Duration	Calories Burned
TOTAL		

Weekly Assessment

Food Intake Summary

DAY 1				
DAY 2				
DAY 3				
DAY 4				
DAY 5				
DAY 6				
DAY 7				
Weekly Total				
Average Daily Intake (Total ÷ 7)				

Did you meet your goals for water and fruit and veggie intake this week?   Yes   No

Exercise Summary

	Type	Duration	Calories Burned
DAY 1			
DAY 2			
DAY 3			
DAY 4			
DAY 5			
DAY 6			
DAY 7			
TOTALS			

Notes & Gold Star Moments

_____
_____
_____
_____
_____
_____
_____
_____
_____
_____
_____

Goals for Next Week

Eating: _____
_____
_____
_____
_____

Exercise: _____
_____
_____

Other: _____
_____

Day/Week	Date	Weight	**235**

Goals for the Day: _____

Morning	Time: __ __:__ __					Mood	Energy
TOTAL							
Afternoon	Time: __ __:__ __						
TOTAL							
Evening	Time: __ __:__ __						
TOTAL							
Snacks							
	Time: __ __:__ __						
	Time: __ __:__ __						
	Time: __ __:__ __						
	Time: __ __:__ __						
TOTAL							
Daily Totals							

Water/Fluid Intake
❑ ❑ ❑ ❑ ❑ ❑ ❑ ❑

Fruits/Vegetables
❑ ❑ ❑ ❑ ❑ ❑ ❑ ❑

Exercise Log

Type	Duration	Calories Burned
TOTAL		

Day/Week	Date	Weight

Goals for the Day: _____

Morning	Time: __ __:__ __						Mood	Energy
TOTAL								
Afternoon	Time: __ __:__ __							
TOTAL								
Evening	Time: __ __:__ __							
TOTAL								
Snacks								
	Time: __ __:__ __							
	Time: __ __:__ __							
	Time: __ __:__ __							
	Time: __ __:__ __							
TOTAL								
Daily Totals								

Water/Fluid Intake
▢ ▢ ▢ ▢ ▢ ▢ ▢ ▢

Fruits/Vegetables
▢ ▢ ▢ ▢ ▢ ▢ ▢ ▢

Exercise Log

Type	Duration	Calories Burned
TOTAL		

Day/Week	Date	Weight	**237**

Goals for the Day: _____

Morning	Time: __ __:__ __					Mood	Energy
TOTAL							
Afternoon	Time: __ __:__ __						
TOTAL							
Evening	Time: __ __:__ __						
TOTAL							
Snacks							
	Time: __ __:__ __						
	Time: __ __:__ __						
	Time: __ __:__ __						
	Time: __ __:__ __						
TOTAL							
Daily Totals							

Water/Fluid Intake
❑ ❑ ❑ ❑ ❑ ❑ ❑ ❑

Fruits/Vegetables
❑ ❑ ❑ ❑ ❑ ❑ ❑ ❑

Exercise Log

Type	Duration	Calories Burned
TOTAL		

238

Day/Week	Date	Weight

Goals for the Day: _____

Morning	Time: __ __:__ __					Mood	Energy
TOTAL							
Afternoon	Time: __ __:__ __						
TOTAL							
Evening	Time: __ __:__ __						
TOTAL							
Snacks							
	Time: __ __:__ __						
	Time: __ __:__ __						
	Time: __ __:__ __						
	Time: __ __:__ __						
TOTAL							
Daily Totals							

Water/Fluid Intake
❑ ❑ ❑ ❑ ❑ ❑ ❑ ❑

Fruits/Vegetables
❑ ❑ ❑ ❑ ❑ ❑ ❑ ❑

Exercise Log

Type	Duration	Calories Burned
TOTAL		

| Day/Week | Date | Weight | **239** |

Goals for the Day: _____

Morning	Time: __ __:__ __					Mood	Energy
TOTAL							

Afternoon	Time: __ __:__ __						
TOTAL							

Evening	Time: __ __:__ __						
TOTAL							

Snacks							
	Time: __ __:__ __						
	Time: __ __:__ __						
	Time: __ __:__ __						
	Time: __ __:__ __						
TOTAL							

| Daily Totals | | | | | | | |

Water/Fluid Intake
❑ ❑ ❑ ❑ ❑ ❑ ❑ ❑

Fruits/Vegetables
❑ ❑ ❑ ❑ ❑ ❑ ❑ ❑

Exercise Log

Type	Duration	Calories Burned
TOTAL		

240

Day/Week	Date	Weight

Goals for the Day: _____

Morning	Time: __ __:__ __					Mood	Energy
TOTAL							
Afternoon	Time: __ __:__ __						
TOTAL							
Evening	Time: __ __:__ __						
TOTAL							
Snacks							
	Time: __ __:__ __						
	Time: __ __:__ __						
	Time: __ __:__ __						
	Time: __ __:__ __						
TOTAL							
Daily Totals							

Water/Fluid Intake
☐ ☐ ☐ ☐ ☐ ☐ ☐ ☐

Fruits/Vegetables
☐ ☐ ☐ ☐ ☐ ☐ ☐ ☐

Exercise Log

Type	Duration	Calories Burned
TOTAL		

Day/Week	Date	Weight

Goals for the Day: _____

Morning	Time: __ __ : __ __					Mood	Energy
TOTAL							
Afternoon	Time: __ __ : __ __						
TOTAL							
Evening	Time: __ __ : __ __						
TOTAL							
Snacks							
	Time: __ __ : __ __						
	Time: __ __ : __ __						
	Time: __ __ : __ __						
	Time: __ __ : __ __						
TOTAL							
Daily Totals							

Water/Fluid Intake
❑ ❑ ❑ ❑ ❑ ❑ ❑ ❑

Fruits/Vegetables
❑ ❑ ❑ ❑ ❑ ❑ ❑ ❑

Exercise Log

Type	Duration	Calories Burned
TOTAL		

Food Intake Summary

DAY 1				
DAY 2				
DAY 3				
DAY 4				
DAY 5				
DAY 6				
DAY 7				
Weekly Total				
Average Daily Intake (Total ÷ 7)				

Did you meet your goals for water and fruit and veggie intake this week?   Yes   No

Exercise Summary

	Type	Duration	Calories Burned
DAY 1			
DAY 2			
DAY 3			
DAY 4			
DAY 5			
DAY 6			
DAY 7			
TOTALS			

Notes & Gold Star Moments

_____
_____
_____
_____
_____
_____
_____
_____
_____
_____

Goals for Next Week

Eating: _____
_____
_____
_____
_____

Exercise: _____
_____
_____

Other: _____

Day/Week	Date	Weight

Goals for the Day: _____

Morning	Time: __ __:__ __					Mood	Energy
TOTAL							
Afternoon	Time: __ __:__ __						
TOTAL							
Evening	Time: __ __:__ __						
TOTAL							
Snacks							
	Time: __ __:__ __						
	Time: __ __:__ __						
	Time: __ __:__ __						
	Time: __ __:__ __						
TOTAL							
Daily Totals							

Water/Fluid Intake
❑ ❑ ❑ ❑ ❑ ❑ ❑ ❑

Fruits/Vegetables
❑ ❑ ❑ ❑ ❑ ❑ ❑ ❑

Exercise Log

Type	Duration	Calories Burned
TOTAL		

244

Goals for the Day: _____

Morning	Time: __ __:__ __					Mood	Energy
TOTAL							
Afternoon	Time: __ __:__ __						
TOTAL							
Evening	Time: __ __:__ __						
TOTAL							
Snacks							
	Time: __ __:__ __						
	Time: __ __:__ __						
	Time: __ __:__ __						
	Time: __ __:__ __						
TOTAL							
Daily Totals							

Water/Fluid Intake
❑ ❑ ❑ ❑ ❑ ❑ ❑ ❑

Fruits/Vegetables
❑ ❑ ❑ ❑ ❑ ❑ ❑ ❑

Exercise Log

Type	Duration	Calories Burned
TOTAL		

Day/Week	Date	Weight

Goals for the Day: _____

Morning	Time: __ __:__ __					Mood	Energy
TOTAL							
Afternoon	Time: __ __:__ __						
TOTAL							
Evening	Time: __ __:__ __						
TOTAL							
Snacks							
	Time: __ __:__ __						
	Time: __ __:__ __						
	Time: __ __:__ __						
	Time: __ __:__ __						
TOTAL							
Daily Totals							

Water/Fluid Intake
☐ ☐ ☐ ☐ ☐ ☐ ☐ ☐

Fruits/Vegetables
☐ ☐ ☐ ☐ ☐ ☐ ☐ ☐

Exercise Log

Type	Duration	Calories Burned
TOTAL		

246

Day/Week	Date	Weight

Goals for the Day: _____

Morning	Time: __ __:__ __					Mood	Energy
TOTAL							
Afternoon	Time: __ __:__ __						
TOTAL							
Evening	Time: __ __:__ __						
TOTAL							
Snacks							
	Time: __ __:__ __						
	Time: __ __:__ __						
	Time: __ __:__ __						
	Time: __ __:__ __						
TOTAL							
Daily Totals							

Water/Fluid Intake
❑ ❑ ❑ ❑ ❑ ❑ ❑ ❑

Fruits/Vegetables
❑ ❑ ❑ ❑ ❑ ❑ ❑ ❑

Exercise Log

Type	Duration	Calories Burned
TOTAL		

Day/Week	Date	Weight

Goals for the Day: _____

Morning	Time: __ __:__ __					Mood	Energy
	TOTAL						
Afternoon	Time: __ __:__ __						
	TOTAL						
Evening	Time: __ __:__ __						
	TOTAL						
Snacks							
	Time: __ __:__ __						
	Time: __ __:__ __						
	Time: __ __:__ __						
	Time: __ __:__ __						
	TOTAL						
Daily Totals							

Water/Fluid Intake
❑ ❑ ❑ ❑ ❑ ❑ ❑ ❑

Fruits/Vegetables
❑ ❑ ❑ ❑ ❑ ❑ ❑ ❑

Exercise Log

Type	Duration	Calories Burned
TOTAL		

Day/Week	Date	Weight

Goals for the Day: _____

Morning	Time: __ __:__ __					Mood	Energy
TOTAL							
Afternoon	Time: __ __:__ __						
TOTAL							
Evening	Time: __ __:__ __						
TOTAL							
Snacks							
	Time: __ __:__ __						
	Time: __ __:__ __						
	Time: __ __:__ __						
	Time: __ __:__ __						
TOTAL							
Daily Totals							

Water/Fluid Intake
☐ ☐ ☐ ☐ ☐ ☐ ☐

Fruits/Vegetables
☐ ☐ ☐ ☐ ☐ ☐ ☐

Exercise Log

Type	Duration	Calories Burned
TOTAL		

Day/Week	Date	Weight	

249

Goals for the Day: _____

Morning	Time: __ __:__ __					Mood	Energy
TOTAL							
Afternoon	Time: __ __:__ __						
TOTAL							
Evening	Time: __ __:__ __						
TOTAL							
Snacks							
	Time: __ __:__ __						
	Time: __ __:__ __						
	Time: __ __:__ __						
	Time: __ __:__ __						
TOTAL							
Daily Totals							

Water/Fluid Intake
❏ ❏ ❏ ❏ ❏ ❏ ❏ ❏

Fruits/Vegetables
❏ ❏ ❏ ❏ ❏ ❏ ❏ ❏

Exercise Log

Type	Duration	Calories Burned
TOTAL		

Weekly Assessment

Food Intake Summary

DAY 1				
DAY 2				
DAY 3				
DAY 4				
DAY 5				
DAY 6				
DAY 7				
Weekly Total				
Average Daily Intake (Total ÷ 7)				

Did you meet your goals for water and fruit and veggie intake this week?   Yes   No

Exercise Summary

	Type	Duration	Calories Burned
DAY 1			
DAY 2			
DAY 3			
DAY 4			
DAY 5			
DAY 6			
DAY 7			
TOTALS			

Notes & Gold Star Moments

Goals for Next Week

Eating:

Exercise:

Other:

Day/Week	Date	Weight

Goals for the Day: _____

Morning Time: __ __:__ __						Mood	Energy
TOTAL							
Afternoon Time: __ __:__ __							
TOTAL							
Evening Time: __ __:__ __							
TOTAL							
Snacks							
Time: __ __:__ __							
Time: __ __:__ __							
Time: __ __:__ __							
Time: __ __:__ __							
TOTAL							
Daily Totals							

Water/Fluid Intake
❑ ❑ ❑ ❑ ❑ ❑ ❑ ❑

Fruits/Vegetables
❑ ❑ ❑ ❑ ❑ ❑ ❑ ❑

Exercise Log

Type	Duration	Calories Burned
TOTAL		

252

Day/Week	Date	Weight

Goals for the Day: _____

Morning	Time: __ __:__ __					Mood	Energy
TOTAL							
Afternoon	Time: __ __:__ __						
TOTAL							
Evening	Time: __ __:__ __						
TOTAL							
Snacks							
	Time: __ __:__ __						
	Time: __ __:__ __						
	Time: __ __:__ __						
	Time: __ __:__ __						
TOTAL							
Daily Totals							

Water/Fluid Intake
☐ ☐ ☐ ☐ ☐ ☐ ☐ ☐

Fruits/Vegetables
☐ ☐ ☐ ☐ ☐ ☐ ☐ ☐

Exercise Log

Type	Duration	Calories Burned
TOTAL		

Day/Week	Date	Weight

Goals for the Day: _____

Morning	Time: __ __:__ __					Mood	Energy
	TOTAL						
Afternoon	Time: __ __:__ __						
	TOTAL						
Evening	Time: __ __:__ __						
	TOTAL						
Snacks							
	Time: __ __:__ __						
	Time: __ __:__ __						
	Time: __ __:__ __						
	Time: __ __:__ __						
	TOTAL						
Daily Totals							

Water/Fluid Intake
☐ ☐ ☐ ☐ ☐ ☐ ☐ ☐

Fruits/Vegetables
☐ ☐ ☐ ☐ ☐ ☐ ☐ ☐

Exercise Log

Type	Duration	Calories Burned
TOTAL		

254

Day/Week	Date	Weight

Goals for the Day: _____

Morning	Time: __ __:__ __						Mood	Energy
TOTAL								
Afternoon	Time: __ __:__ __							
TOTAL								
Evening	Time: __ __:__ __							
TOTAL								
Snacks								
	Time: __ __:__ __							
	Time: __ __:__ __							
	Time: __ __:__ __							
	Time: __ __:__ __							
TOTAL								
Daily Totals								

Water/Fluid Intake
❏ ❏ ❏ ❏ ❏ ❏ ❏ ❏

Fruits/Vegetables
❏ ❏ ❏ ❏ ❏ ❏ ❏ ❏

Exercise Log

Type	Duration	Calories Burned
TOTAL		

Day/Week	Date	Weight

Goals for the Day: _____

Morning Time: __ __:__ __						Mood	Energy
TOTAL							
Afternoon Time: __ __:__ __							
TOTAL							
Evening Time: __ __:__ __							
TOTAL							
Snacks							
Time: __ __:__ __							
Time: __ __:__ __							
Time: __ __:__ __							
Time: __ __:__ __							
TOTAL							
Daily Totals							

Water/Fluid Intake   *Fruits/Vegetables*
▢▢▢▢▢▢▢▢   ▢▢▢▢▢▢▢▢

Exercise Log

Type	Duration	Calories Burned
TOTAL		

Day/Week	Date	Weight

Goals for the Day: _____

Morning	Time: __ __:__ __						Mood	Energy
TOTAL								
Afternoon	Time: __ __:__ __							
TOTAL								
Evening	Time: __ __:__ __							
TOTAL								
Snacks								
	Time: __ __:__ __							
	Time: __ __:__ __							
	Time: __ __:__ __							
	Time: __ __:__ __							
TOTAL								
Daily Totals								

Water/Fluid Intake
☐ ☐ ☐ ☐ ☐ ☐ ☐ ☐

Fruits/Vegetables
☐ ☐ ☐ ☐ ☐ ☐ ☐ ☐

Exercise Log

Type	Duration	Calories Burned
TOTAL		

Day/Week	Date	Weight	**257**

Goals for the Day: _____

Morning	Time: __ __:__ __						Mood	Energy
TOTAL								
Afternoon	Time: __ __:__ __							
TOTAL								
Evening	Time: __ __:__ __							
TOTAL								
Snacks								
	Time: __ __:__ __							
	Time: __ __:__ __							
	Time: __ __:__ __							
	Time: __ __:__ __							
TOTAL								
Daily Totals								

Water/Fluid Intake
❑ ❑ ❑ ❑ ❑ ❑ ❑ ❑

Fruits/Vegetables
❑ ❑ ❑ ❑ ❑ ❑ ❑ ❑

Exercise Log

Type	**Duration**	**Calories Burned**
TOTAL		

Food Intake Summary

DAY 1				
DAY 2				
DAY 3				
DAY 4				
DAY 5				
DAY 6				
DAY 7				
Weekly Total				
Average Daily Intake (Total ÷ 7)				

Did you meet your goals for water and fruit and veggie intake this week?   Yes   No

Exercise Summary

	Type	Duration	Calories Burned
DAY 1			
DAY 2			
DAY 3			
DAY 4			
DAY 5			
DAY 6			
DAY 7			
TOTALS			

Notes & Gold Star Moments

_____
_____
_____
_____
_____
_____
_____
_____
_____
_____
_____
_____

Goals for Next Week

Eating: _____
_____
_____
_____
_____

Exercise: _____
_____
_____

Other: _____
_____

Apple & Macs

iPad For Dummies
978-0-470-58027-1

iPhone For Dummies,
4th Edition
978-0-470-87870-5

MacBook For
Dummies, 3rd Edition
978-0-470-76918-8

Mac OS X Snow
Leopard For
Dummies
978-0-470-43543-4

Business

Bookkeeping For
Dummies
978-0-7645-9848-7

Job Interviews
For Dummies,
3rd Edition
978-0-470-17748-8

Resumes For
Dummies,
5th Edition
978-0-470-08037-5

Starting an
Online Business
For Dummies,
6th Edition
978-0-470-60210-2

Stock Investing
For Dummies,
3rd Edition
978-0-470-40114-9

Successful
Time Management
For Dummies
978-0-470-29034-7

Computer Hardware

BlackBerry
For Dummies,
4th Edition
978-0-470-60700-8

Computers For
Seniors
For Dummies,
2nd Edition
978-0-470-53483-0

PCs For Dummies,
Windows 7 Edition
978-0-470-46542-4

Laptops For
Dummies,
4th Edition
978-0-470-57829-2

Cooking & Entertaining

Cooking Basics
For Dummies,
3rd Edition
978-0-7645-7206-7

Wine For Dummies,
4th Edition
978-0-470-04579-4

Diet & Nutrition

Dieting For Dummies,
2nd Edition
978-0-7645-4149-0

Nutrition For
Dummies,
4th Edition
978-0-471-79868-2

Weight Training
For Dummies,
3rd Edition
978-0-471-76845-6

Digital Photography

Digital SLR Cameras
& Photography For
Dummies, 3rd Edition
978-0-470-46606-3

Photoshop Elements 8
For Dummies
978-0-470-52967-6

Gardening

Gardening Basics
For Dummies
978-0-470-03749-2

Organic Gardening
For Dummies,
2nd Edition
978-0-470-43067-5

Green/Sustainable

Raising Chickens
For Dummies
978-0-470-46544-8

Green Cleaning
For Dummies
978-0-470-39106-8

Health

Diabetes For
Dummies,
3rd Edition
978-0-470-27086-8

Food Allergies
For Dummies
978-0-470-09584-3

Living Gluten-Free
For Dummies,
2nd Edition
978-0-470-58589-4

Hobbies/General

Chess For Dummies,
2nd Edition
978-0-7645-8404-6

Drawing
Cartoons & Comics
For Dummies
978-0-470-42683-8

Knitting For Dummies,
2nd Edition
978-0-470-28747-7

Organizing
For Dummies
978-0-7645-5300-4

Su Doku For
Dummies
978-0-470-01892-7

Home Improvement

Home Maintenance
For Dummies,
2nd Edition
978-0-470-43063-7

Home Theater
For Dummies,
3rd Edition
978-0-470-41189-6

Living the
Country Lifestyle
All-in-One
For Dummies
978-0-470-43061-3

Solar Power Your
Home
For Dummies,
2nd Edition
978-0-470-59678-4

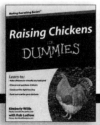

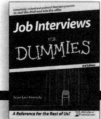

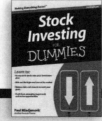

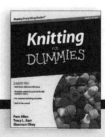

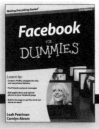
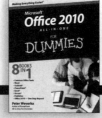
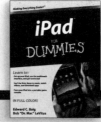
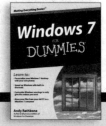